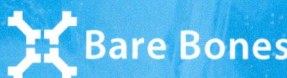

Bare Bones

Anaesthesia

A GUIDE FOR MEDICAL STUDENTS

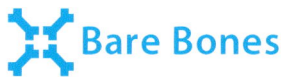 **Bare Bones**

Anaesthesia

A GUIDE FOR MEDICAL STUDENTS

Adam Arshad, BSc (Hons), MBChB (Hons), PgCert (MedEd), MRCSEd, FHEA
ST2 Trauma and Orthopaedics Academic Clinical Fellow – University Hospitals
Coventry and Warwickshire

Pooja Devani, iBsc (Hons), MBChB
ST3 Paediatrics Academic Clinical Fellow – University Hospitals Leicester

Sonika Sethi, iBsc (Hons), MBBS, MRCP
ST3 Gastroenterology Academic Clinical Fellow – Chelsea and Westminster Hospital

Arjuna Thakker, BSc, MBChB, MRCSEd, PgCert (MedEd)
CT1 Plastic Surgery – The James Cook University Hospital

Nicholas Marsden, BSc, MBBS, PgCert (MedEd), FRCA, MSc
ST7 Anaesthetic Trainee, West Midlands Deanery

Simran Minhas, MBBS, FRCA, PgCert Keele (Clinical Leadership)
Consultant Anaesthetist, Royal Orthopaedic Hospital Birmingham

Scion

© **Scion Publishing Ltd, 2024**

First published 2024

A CIP catalogue record for this book is available from the British Library.

ISBN 9781911510987

Scion Publishing Limited

The Old Hayloft, Vantage Business Park, Bloxham Road, Banbury OX16 9UX, UK

www.scionpublishing.com

Important Note from the Publisher

The information contained within this book was obtained by Scion Publishing Ltd from sources believed by us to be reliable. However, while every effort has been made to ensure its accuracy, no responsibility for loss or injury whatsoever occasioned to any person acting or refraining from action as a result of information contained herein can be accepted by the authors or publishers.

Readers are reminded that medicine is a constantly evolving science and while the authors and publishers have ensured that all dosages, applications and practices are based on current indications, there may be specific practices which differ between communities. You should always follow the guidelines laid down by the manufacturers of specific products and the relevant authorities in the country in which you are practising.

Although every effort has been made to ensure that all owners of copyright material have been acknowledged in this publication, we would be pleased to acknowledge in subsequent reprints or editions any omissions brought to our attention.

Registered names, trademarks, etc. used in this book, even when not marked as such, are not to be considered unprotected by law.

Cover design by Andrew Magee Design
Typeset by Evolution Design & Digital Ltd (Kent)
Printed in the UK

Last digit is the print number: 10 9 8 7 6 5 4 3 2

CHAPTER 1

Principles of anaesthesia

1.1	General anaesthesia – the basics	4
1.2	Induction agents	5
	1.2.1 Intravenous and intramuscular induction agents	5
	1.2.2 Inhaled induction agents	8
1.3	Analgesics	11
1.4	Neuromuscular blockers	13
	1.4.1 Depolarising agents	15
	1.4.2 Non-depolarising agents	16

An anaesthetist is a postgraduate doctor whose primary role involves the care of patients in the operating theatre.

The word anaesthesia derives from the Greek word *anaesthetos*, meaning without sensation – and in the operating theatre, the role of the anaesthetist is to reduce or completely remove the sensation experienced by the patient.

There are three broad types of anaesthesia:

- General anaesthesia (GA)
- Regional anaesthesia
- Local anaesthesia.

Each of these is a different method to reduce a patient's sensation during a procedure and each can be used in isolation, or in combination with another (when used in combination, we call this multimodal anaesthesia).

General anaesthesia

This is your classic 'falling asleep' anaesthesia. When we deliver an anaesthetic drug that induces GA (these drugs are called GA agents or hypnotics), the patient enters unconsciousness (or hypnosis) that can be reversed. The reasons this occurs are still being elucidated. When delivery of a GA agent is stopped, the patient will emerge with no recollection of the events (amnesia).

When conducting GA, we may also need to:

- deliver analgesics (pain relief medication) to reduce the surgical stress response (see the *Key notes* box below)
- potentially give a muscle relaxant (if required for the procedure) to help the surgeon access certain body areas (without a muscle relaxant, the tone of the muscles can make the surgical procedure difficult).

KEY NOTES

What is the surgical stress response?

This is the systemic response of the body to surgical injury. It involves activation of the sympathetic nervous and endocrine systems, which promotes metabolism and catabolism. These are normal body responses if an injury is sustained. Typical changes, as part of the surgical stress response, include increases in:

- adrenaline
- cortisol
- glucagon (but reductions in insulin)
- renin
- growth hormone.

We want to prevent these responses occurring mid-surgery, because they could lead to harmful cardiovascular and metabolic changes (e.g. adrenaline release causing profound tachycardia).

These three components (**hypnotics**, **analgesics** and **muscle relaxants**) are known as the triad of anaesthesia, and need to be considered every time we conduct GA.

Regional anaesthesia

Regional anaesthesia (see *Chapter 7*) involves interrupting nerve signals from a single nerve or groups of nerves, without inducing hypnosis (as is seen with GA). When you see individuals undergoing surgery, but awake, that's regional anaesthesia!

Local anaesthesia

While regional anaesthesia blocks specific nerves/nerve groups, local anaesthesia blocks nerve transmission from smaller nerve endings to a superficial location for a specific procedure, e.g. a skin laceration requiring suturing. See *Chapter 6* for more on local anaesthesia.

1.1 General anaesthesia – the basics

We will first cover general anaesthesia. In the later chapters, we will then discuss regional and local anaesthesia.

When delivering GA there are three key medications that we can provide. As discussed, these are known as the triad of anaesthesia:

- **GA agents** – also called hypnotics, these are what put the patient into the reversible, unconscious state. The agent itself can be administered intravenously (IV), intramuscularly (IM), or as an inhaled drug.
- **Analgesics** – these reduce the patient's pain sensation, to reduce the surgical stress response.
- **Muscle relaxants** (or neuromuscular blockers) – to relax the muscles.

It may not always be necessary to provide all three types of medication, but consideration to all three is required when conducting GA.

There are generally three key stages in the process of administering a general anaesthesia:

1. Induction – getting the patient to sleep
2. Maintenance – keeping the patient asleep during the operation
3. Emergence – waking the patient up at the end of the procedure.

We will initially cover the theory of the medications and preparing a patient for anaesthesia, before going into the steps of induction, maintenance and emergence in *Chapter 3*.

KEY NOTES

How do GA agents work?
The exact mechanism of hypnotic agents is poorly understood. It's considered to be secondary to agonist action on the neurotransmitter receptor $GABA_A$ in the central nervous system (CNS). GABA (gamma aminobutyric acid) has an inhibitory effect on the formation of action potentials.

1.2 Induction agents

1.2.1 Intravenous and intramuscular induction agents

Propofol

Formula: $C_{12}H_{18}O$

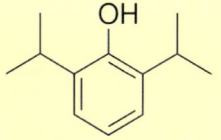

General information: propofol is the most commonly used IV induction agent. Propofol is stored in glass vials at 1% or 2% concentration. It has a characteristic white colour, as the medication is prepared in a lipid emulsion (see *Figure 1.1*).

Uses:

1. Propofol is used at induction and in the maintenance of GA.
2. It has anticonvulsant properties and can be used in managing status epilepticus.

Advantages:

- Propofol provides a fast induction and offset of GA, due to its short half-life.
- Therefore recovery from propofol is quick (because of its short half-life).
- Propofol suppresses the laryngeal reflexes, allowing the insertion of airway devices.

Disadvantages:

- Propofol can cause pain on injection, particularly if administered into small veins. A small dose of lidocaine in the same vein can mitigate this side-effect.
- Bolus injection causes a fall in systemic vascular resistance, which may cause hypotension in clinically unstable patients.
- Continued administration of propofol can lead to 'propofol infusion syndrome' (when over 4 mg/kg/hr is administered for prolonged periods, e.g. in ICU). This occurs in 1% of all

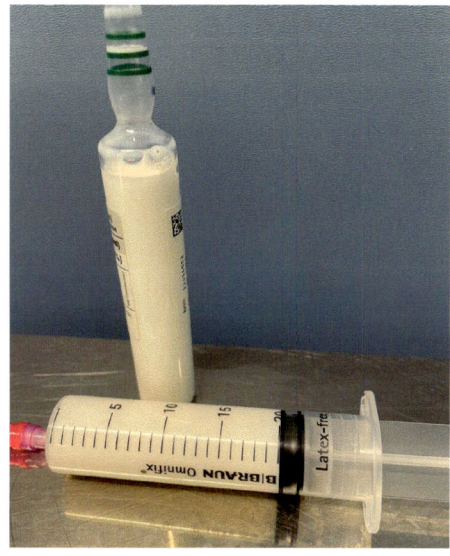

Figure 1.1: A syringe and bottle of 1% propofol – note its characteristic white colour.

ICU patients who are sedated with propofol. In this syndrome, patients experience:

- metabolic acidosis
- cardiac dysfunction
- rhabdomyolysis
- renal failure
- green urine (secondary to the metabolites of propofol).

Thiopental sodium (also known as thiopentone)

Formula: $C_{11}H_{17}N_2NaO_2S$

General information: this is a short-acting hypnotic agent (group name: barbiturates), which rapidly induces GA.

Uses:

1. Used IV, for induction of GA only. An alternative agent is required for maintenance anaesthesia.
2. Occasionally used as an infusion on ICU in management of status epilepticus.

Advantages:

- Thiopental sodium has a rapid onset of action, with the patient rendered unconscious within 30 seconds of administration. Its effects last 4–7 minutes (for this reason it was initially the drug of choice for induction in emergency settings until experience with propofol was gained).

Disadvantages:

- Rapid administration reduces cardiac contractility and decreases systemic vascular resistance, which can result in profound hypotension.
- Thiopental sodium is administered for induction GA **only** (and not for maintenance). Prolonged infusions of thiopental sodium accumulate in the tissue compartment, meaning that GA is maintained even after the infusion has stopped. This results in a longer wake-up time and can increase the risk of adverse side-effects.
- Thiopental sodium is contraindicated in patients diagnosed with porphyria, as it can trigger an acute porphyria attack.
- Thiopental sodium does not suppress the airway reflexes (unlike propofol).
- Thiopental sodium does not have a proven analgesic effect (unlike propofol which does, and therefore provides some pain relief, as well as hypnosis, to the patient).

Ketamine

Formula: $C_{13}H_{16}CINO$

General information: ketamine is a phencyclidine derivative, which is the drug of abuse commonly known as Special K. Ketamine is used as an induction agent in emergency settings as it has favourable cardiovascular effects. It also has very strong analgesic properties, and so is used for both acute and chronic analgesia.

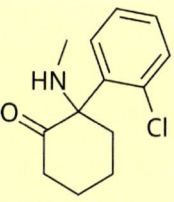

Unlike other hypnotic agents, ketamine can be administered either IV or IM.

Uses:

1. Low doses of ketamine are used as sedation for procedures such as burns dressing changes.
2. Ketamine can be used for induction of GA or in combination with other induction agents.
3. Low dose infusions can be used in complicated pain cases, or for surgery where pain control may be challenging.

Advantages:

- Ketamine has superior analgesic properties to other IV hypnotic agents.
- Its cardiovascular stability makes it useful in cardiovascularly unstable patients (due to sympathomimetic effects).

Disadvantages:

- Induction of anaesthesia is not as rapid as with propofol or thiopental sodium.
- Patients can develop an emergence phenomenon during the recovery period after receiving ketamine; this can include hallucinations, alterations in mood state and vivid dreams. Administering benzodiazepines, both as a premedication and after the procedure, reduces the incidence of these adverse effects.
- Caution must be exercised when providing ketamine in the following patient groups, as ketamine is associated with psychological disturbance, raised intracranial and intraocular pressure:
  - acute or chronic alcohol intoxication
  - raised intracranial pressure
  - raised intraocular pressure
  - psychosis.
- High dose chronic use is known to have detrimental effects on the urinary tract (known as ketamine bladder).

1.2.2 Inhaled induction agents

Inhalational GA agents are also referred to as 'volatile agents'. They are predominantly used in the maintenance of anaesthesia, but patients can be induced using these agents (a gas induction).

These agents are stored as a liquid, and require a vaporiser to safely deliver them to the patient. They readily turn from a liquid to a vapour at room temperature.

KEY NOTES

What is minimum alveolar concentration?

This is a key term to learn. In the abbreviated form of minimum alveolar concentration, MAC_a, the 'a' signifies atmospheric pressure. It is the concentration of the inhalational agent that is required to inhibit a physical response in 50% of patients when receiving a standardised painful stimulus.

MAC_{50} is influenced by several factors, including:

- anxiety (increases MAC)
- age (MAC is higher in infants, lower in the elderly)
- hypothermia (decreases MAC)
- hypotension (decreases MAC)
- pregnancy (decreases MAC)
- depressed level of consciousness or cognitive/neurodegenerative changes, e.g. dementia (decreases MAC).

MAC values aid an anaesthetist gauging the amount of inhaled GA agent to be used. They do not influence our choice of inhaled GA agent – but help us determine the amount we need to provide. A higher MAC_a value means more volume of inhaled GA is required to provide GA.

Isoflurane

MAC_a value: 1.15% (a signifies atmospheric pressure)

Formula: $C_3H_2ClF_5O$

General information: isoflurane (and sevoflurane – see below) is from a group of anaesthetic agents called 'halogenated ethers'. Both are colourless but have distinct odours.

Uses:

1. Maintenance of GA.
2. Can be used for induction GA, but sevoflurane is preferred (see reasons below).

Advantages:
- Isoflurane is a cheap inhalational agent which has a good safety profile.
- Rapid achievement of GA.

Disadvantages:
- Upper airway irritant, therefore is not the ideal agent for gas induction.
- Slower recovery from anaesthesia when compared with other inhalation GA agents.
- Drops systemic vascular resistance, resulting in hypotension.
- Theoretically can cause 'cardiac steal'. This is a phenomenon where myocardial perfusion is reduced by coronary artery vasodilatation.

Sevoflurane

MAC$_a$ value: 2.0%

Formula: $C_4H_3F_7O$

General information: sevoflurane is currently the most frequently used inhalation agent. It has an excellent safety record.

F_3C O F
CF_3

Uses:
1. Sevoflurane is used in both induction and maintenance of GA.

Advantages:
- Sevoflurane is less irritating to the upper airway than isoflurane and well tolerated when used for gas inductions (i.e. instead of an IV induction agent).
- Sevoflurane has a faster onset and offset than isoflurane.

Disadvantages:
- Sevoflurane lowers systemic vascular resistance, which may result in hypotension.
- Theoretically sevoflurane can cause 'cardiac steal'. This is a phenomenon where myocardial perfusion is reduced by coronary artery vasodilatation, altering regional blood flow.
- A metabolite of isoflurane and sevoflurane, called compound A, can cause nephrotoxicity. However, studies further detailing this are lacking.

Halothane

MAC$_a$ value: 0.8%

Formula: $C_2HBrClF_3$

General information: halothane is a colourless, odourless gas. It is no longer used as ~1 in 10 000 patients receiving halothane develop hepatitis, with a 30–70% mortality rate. However, it is still used extensively in developing countries around the world.

1.3 Analgesics

Analgesia will be administered to the patient preoperatively, perioperatively and postoperatively.

Preoperative analgesia is considered to reduce the surgical stress response of the patient in the operating theatre.

Perioperative analgesia reduces the surgical stress response and pain relief requirements after surgery.

It is important that we always consider analgesia, and provide it if required. This is why analgesia forms one part of the triad of GA (as discussed in *Section 1.1*).

For preoperative and perioperative analgesia, we tend to simply provide patients with paracetamol + ibuprofen + opiates. If the patient is undergoing major surgery where significant pain is anticipated, more complex forms of analgesia, e.g. peripheral nerve blocks, can be used. Peripheral nerve blocks are described in *Section 7.1*.

Postoperative analgesia helps patients control pain from the surgical procedure and allows them to start rehabilitation (e.g. walking, other movement). The World Health Organization (WHO) pain relief ladder[1] provides a framework for prescribing postoperative analgesia (see *Figure 1.2*). Typical doses and examples of medications are provided in *Table 1.1*. It should be noted that this ladder is to be tailored to a patient's medical history (e.g. to not prescribe non-steroidal anti-inflammatory drugs (NSAIDs) in renal dysfunction).

Table 1.1: Doses and examples of medications within the WHO pain ladder

Medications	Examples and maximum doses (adults)
Step 1	
Non-opioids	Paracetamol 1 g PO/IV QDS Ibuprofen 400 mg PO TDS
Adjuvants	Bandages, braces, deep heat, massages
Step 2	
Weak opioids	Codeine 30 mg QDS or Dihydrocodeine 30 mg up to 6× a day
Adjuvants	Pregabalin, gabapentin*

Step 3	
Strong opioids	Tramadol 100 mg PO QDS Oramorph (initially 10 mg every 4 hours) Patient-controlled analgesia (PCA) (described in *Section 7.3.1*)

*For neuropathic pain only. Doses depend on previous exposure and to be titrated accordingly.

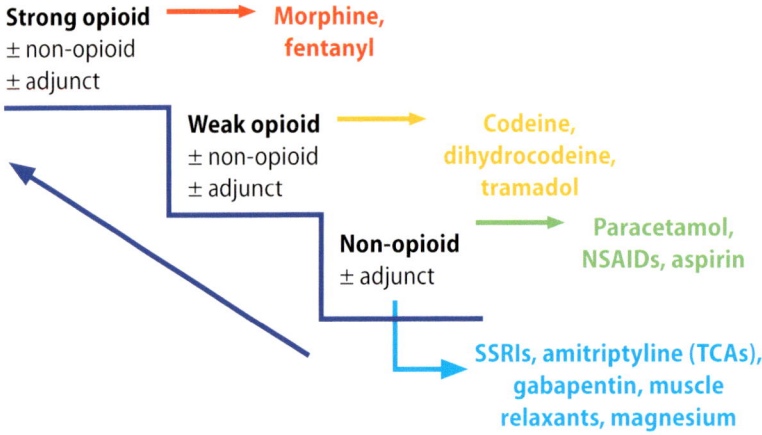

Figure 1.2: The World Health Organization Pain Ladder.

1.4 Neuromuscular blockers

Drugs that cause reversible skeletal muscle paralysis are known as neuromuscular blocking drugs (NMBDs). They are sometimes referred to as muscle relaxants, but it is important to remember that they work at the interface between nerves and muscles – the neuromuscular junction – *not on the muscles themselves*.

NMBDs are a group of compounds that competitively inhibit the nicotinic acetylcholine receptor (nAChR) at the neuromuscular junction.

An NMBD is used in GA in the following circumstances:

- If the patient requires endotracheal intubation – this is discussed further in *Section 4.3*.
- Patient, surgical or anaesthetic factors require muscle paralysis, e.g. prolonged surgery, abdominal surgery, surgery in the prone position and patients with high body mass index (BMI). Without muscle paralysis, the tone of the muscles makes surgery in these individuals very difficult.

NMBDs are divided into two groups: **depolarising** and **non-depolarising agents**.

Depolarising NMBDs act as agonists at the nAChR, to initially cause depolarisation, muscle contractions (called fasciculations) and then temporary inhibition of the nAChR.

Non-depolarising NMBDs act as an antagonist at the nAChR. Therefore their binding does not cause initial fasciculations.

In current clinical practice, non-depolarising agents are more commonly used.

Before discussing common neuromuscular blockers, let's consider the process of impulse transmission at the neuromuscular junction (NMJ) (*see Figure 1.3*).

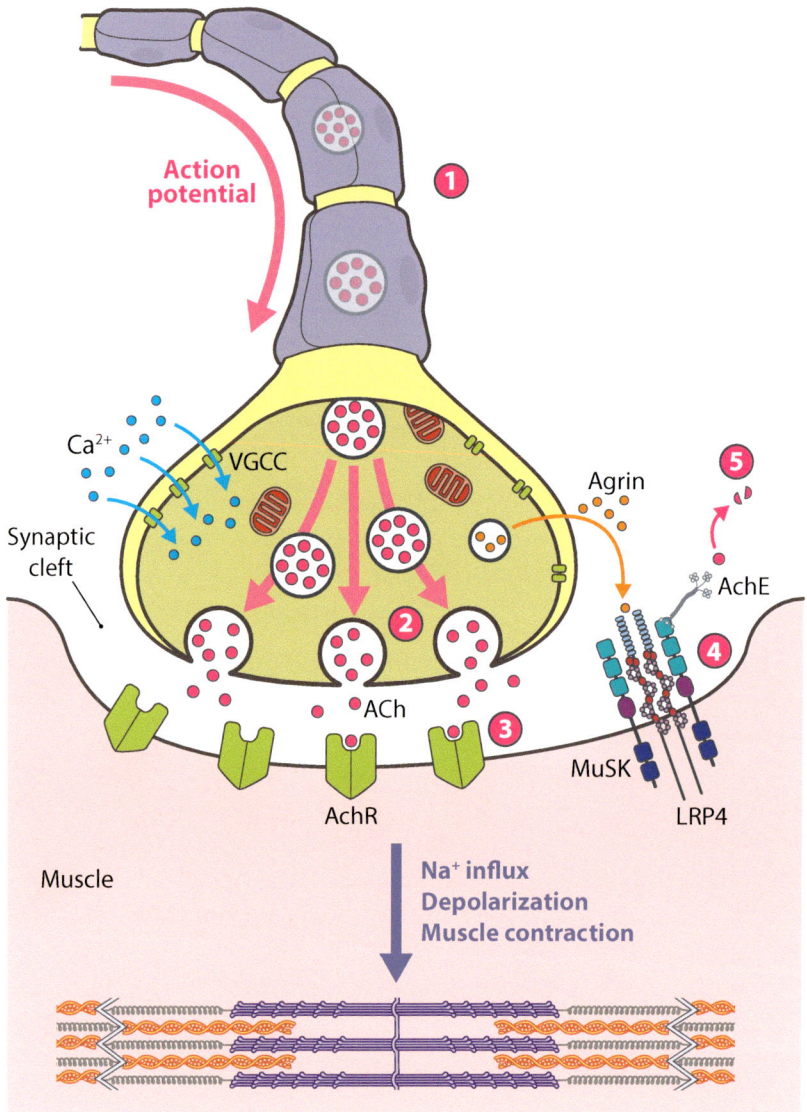

Figure 1.3: Transmission of the nerve impulse at the neuromuscular junction.
At ① the action potential (AP) arrives at the presynaptic nerve. The depolarisation of the presynaptic nerve causes the opening of the presynaptic voltage-gated Ca^{2+} channels; this results in the influx of Ca^{2+}.
At ② the influx of Ca^{2+} causes vesicles of acetylcholine (ACh) to fuse the presynaptic neuron membrane, releasing the ACh into the synaptic space.
At ③ ACh binds to nicotinic receptors located at the postsynaptic terminal, resulting in the influx of Na^+ into the postsynaptic neuron.
This depolarisation at ④ results in the release of Ca^{2+} from the sarcoplasmic reticulum, which triggers muscle contraction.
ACh in the synaptic space ⑤ is degraded by acetylcholinesterase (AChE).

1.4.1 Depolarising agents

Depolarising NMBDs are agonists at the nAChR at the NMJ. The agent binds to the receptor, causing contractions (fasciculations). It then remains in position at the receptor, preventing repolarisation.

Suxamethonium

Formula: $C_{14}H_{30}Cl_2N_2O_4$

General information: the only depolarising NMBD in use is suxamethonium. As suxamethonium diffuses away from the nAChR, it is broken down by an enzyme called plasma cholinesterase.

Uses:

1. Suxamethonium is reserved for a specific circumstance in GA called rapid sequence induction (RSI; discussed in *Section 3.1.1*).
2. It is unusual to use suxamethonium in elective surgery. It is a very short-acting muscle relaxant reserved for patients who are not fully starved or have a difficult airway to manage. It provides intubating conditions within 30 seconds of administration, but usually wears off within a few minutes.

Advantages:

- Fast, reproducible muscle paralysis in order to prevent aspiration events and the possibility of hypoxia in a compromised airway situation.

However, rocuronium (see over), a newer non-depolarising NMBD, offers similar properties and has a targeted reversal agent and no adverse consequences of fasciculation. This drug is taking the place of suxamethonium in clinical practice.

Disadvantages:

- Suxamethonium opens the nAChR, which results in an increase in serum potassium (the increase can be 0.5 mmol/L). For this reason, suxamethonium is contraindicated in patients who have a burn or crush injury, patients with pre-existing hyperkalaemia, or patients with denervating conditions.
- A rare but potentially fatal complication can be malignant hyperthermia, which is also possible after administering inhaled GA anaesthetic agents (see *Section 5.7*).
- Suxamethonium apnoea is a familial condition in which individuals are unable to metabolise suxamethonium (discussed in further detail in *Section 5.8*). This leads to prolonged muscle paralysis in the postoperative period.
- Suxamethonium raises intraocular and intracerebral pressure and so it is contraindicated in patients with glaucoma or head injury.

1.4.2 Non-depolarising agents

Non-depolarising agents are competitive antagonists at the nAChR. By completely blocking the nAChR, they cause muscle paralysis without resulting in the initial muscle contractions (fasciculations) seen with depolarising agents.

There are two groups of non-depolarising agent: amino-steroid based drugs and benzylisoquinoliniums.

Rocuronium

Formula: $C_{32}H_{53}BrN_2O_4$

General information: rocuronium is an amino-steroid drug.

Uses:

1. Rocuronium is used in elective and emergency GA due to the advantages listed below.

Advantages:

- Rocuronium has a speed of onset and duration of action that is dose-dependent. Intubating conditions can be achieved quickly (approx. 90 seconds) in an emergency with a large dose (1.2 mg/kg).
- Rocuronium is rapidly reversed by sugammadex (see *Key notes* box below). This is useful if there are complications with oxygenation on induction, e.g. failed intubation. The dose of sugammadex required depends on the dose (mg/kg) of rocuronium given.

Disadvantages:

- Rocuronium is associated with a higher incidence of anaphylaxis than other NMBDs (rate of 1:3500).

KEY NOTES

What is sugammadex?

Sugammadex is a medication for the reversal of neuromuscular blockade by rocuronium. Administered intravenously, its results are rapid and provide predictable recovery of muscular function.

Atracurium

Formula: $C_{65}H_{82}N_2O_{18}S_2$

General information: it is a part of the benzylisoquinolinium group.

Uses:

1. Atracurium is used for medium duration muscle relaxation and in patients with kidney or liver failure. Atracurium is 40% metabolised by 'Hofmann elimination' which is the spontaneous fragmentation of atracurium, occurring at body temperature and pH. The remaining 60% is metabolised via ester hydrolysis by non-specific esterases in the body. These two routes are independent of renal and hepatic function.

Advantages:

- Atracurium pharmacokinetics are more predictable in patients with renal and hepatic failure.

Disadvantages:

- Atracurium causes the release of histamine that may result in:
  - cutaneous flushing
  - hypotension and reflex tachycardia
  - bronchospasm.
- Atracurium is not used in RSI settings because increasing the dose does not increase its speed of onset. Three minutes are required after administration in order to reliably provide muscle relaxation (see *Section 3.1.1* on RSI).

KEY NOTES

Which neuromuscular blockers do we provide to patients with myasthenia gravis?

Myasthenia gravis is an autoimmune condition where IgG antibodies attack nAChR at the neuromuscular junction. This impairs neuromuscular transmission and the patient has a reduced ability to voluntarily use their muscles.

This creates an issue when choosing an appropriate medication for neuromuscular blockade. Generally, patients with myasthenia gravis are less susceptible to depolarising neuromuscular blockers such as suxamethonium. This is because they already have a limited number of functional nAChR.

These patients are **more susceptible** to non-depolarising neuromuscular blockers. A small amount of the agent will block the limited number of nAChR that are present.

If neuromuscular blockade is required in a patient with myasthenia gravis, very small amounts of a non-depolarising agent (e.g. rocuronium) are required because such patients are more sensitive. All patients with myasthenia gravis should be warned of potential postoperative respiratory distress or loss of airway protection after emergence from GA due to prolonged muscle paralysis.

All such patients should be considered for high dependency unit (HDU)/ICU postoperatively due to an increased risk of adverse events, e.g. inadequate ventilation secondary to reduced power.

CHAPTER 2

Preoperative assessment and planning

2.1	A – the Anaesthetic history	21
2.2	A – Airway planning	23
2.3	B – Bloods and investigations	25
	2.3.1 Patient fitness	25
	2.3.2 Surgical grade	25
	2.3.3 Other investigations	29
2.4	C – Comorbidities: medication management	32
	2.4.1 Diabetic medications	32
	2.4.2 Steroids	33
	2.4.3 Anticoagulation and antiplatelet medications	35
	2.4.4 Oral contraceptive pill	36
	2.4.5 Anti-epileptic and Parkinson's medications	36
2.5	D – Drugs to provide	37
	2.5.1 Analgesia	37
	2.5.2 Antacids	37
	2.5.3 Anxiolytics	37
2.6	D – DVT/VTE prophylaxis	38
	2.6.1 Risk assessment	39
	2.6.2 Methods of providing VTE prophylaxis	40
2.7	E – Entering surgical recovery	43
2.8	F – Fasting	44
2.9	Safety – conducting the WHO surgical checklist	45
	2.9.1 Prior to induction – sign-in	45
	2.9.2 Before skin incision – time out	45
	2.9.3 Before the patient leaves the operating room – sign-out	46

Preoperative assessment

Preoperative assessments are conducted to ensure surgery/anaesthesia is performed safely. All elective surgery patients should have a preoperative screening, conducted in a multidisciplinary clinic called a preoperative assessment clinic (POAC). Preoperative assessment is usually conducted three months prior to the elective surgery date. This allows for medication management and optimisation of the patient's comorbidities. In emergency settings, patients will be reviewed by an anaesthetist immediately prior to their surgery and a thorough evaluation of perioperative risk will determine how and when surgery/anaesthesia are conducted.

Assessment on the day of surgery

All patients (whether elective or emergency) will receive a further assessment on the day of surgery.

Through these two assessments, an anaesthetist will ensure that the patient is safe to be anaesthetised and any difficulties are appropriately planned for. The key features that they will consider during these assessments can be remembered easily in the following way: ABCDEF (see *Figure 2.1*):

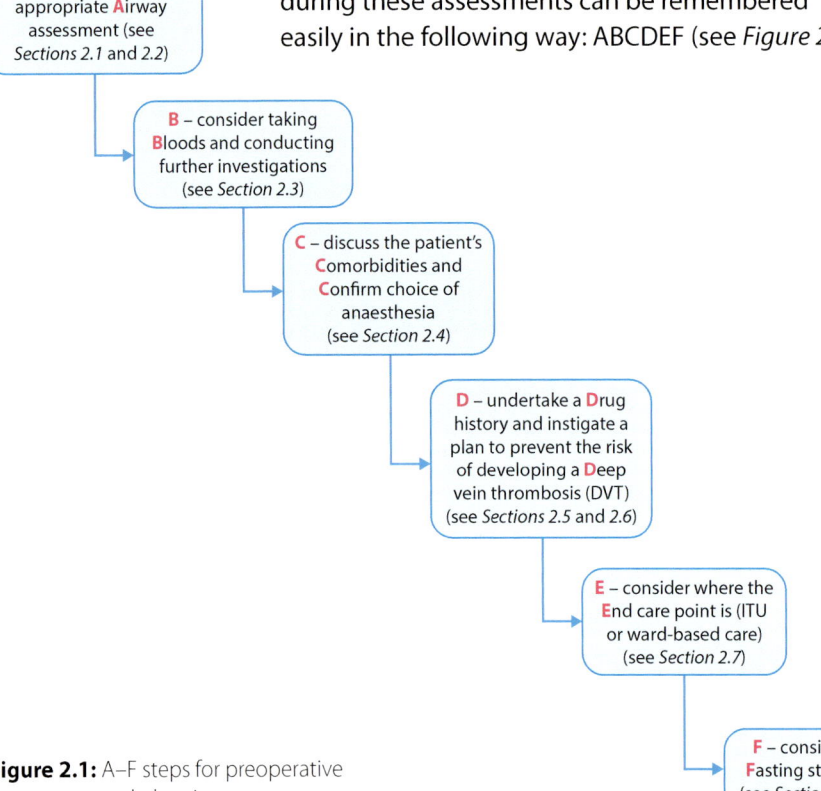

A – take an **A**naesthetic history from the patient and plan their appropriate **A**irway assessment (see *Sections 2.1* and *2.2*)

B – consider taking **B**loods and conducting further investigations (see *Section 2.3*)

C – discuss the patient's **C**omorbidities and **C**onfirm choice of anaesthesia (see *Section 2.4*)

D – undertake a **D**rug history and instigate a plan to prevent the risk of developing a **D**eep vein thrombosis (DVT) (see *Sections 2.5* and *2.6*)

E – consider where the **E**nd care point is (ITU or ward-based care) (see *Section 2.7*)

F – consider **F**asting status (see *Section 2.8*)

Figure 2.1: A–F steps for preoperative assessment and planning.

2.1 A – the Anaesthetic history

An integral aspect of the preoperative assessment is taking a full medical history. It leads to an understanding of the patient's present physical health, previous experience of anaesthesia, current medications, and an evaluation of their potential risk of having complications from anaesthesia/surgery.

The structure of the anaesthetic history is identical to that of a clinical history, with the addition of a section on the patient's past anaesthetic experience. This involves a discussion and review of documentation from previous anaesthesia that the patient has received.

STRUCTURE OF THE ANAESTHETIC HISTORY

1. History of presenting complaint
- Confirm patient procedure and site

2. Medical history
Which medical conditions does the patient have? The following in particular are worthy of further consideration:
- Cardiovascular diseases
- Respiratory diseases (e.g. asthma, chronic obstructive pulmonary disease)
- Renal diseases (e.g. chronic kidney disease), liver diseases, haematological diseases
- Endocrine diseases
- Neurological diseases.

Determining a patient's comorbidities helps ascertain their fitness for surgery and the type of anaesthesia that may be appropriate.

3. Surgical history
- Any previous operations?
  - if yes, where was the operation and why was it required?

4. Anaesthetic history
- Any previous anaesthesia?
  - if yes, were there any complications from the anaesthesia?
  - previous admission to intensive care unit (ICU) and the reasons for this.

5. Drug history
- Current medication list with doses; there are certain drugs which must be altered preoperatively (see *Section 2.4* for the common drug changes that we undertake)
- Ask about any drug allergies and the type of allergic reaction experienced.

Diabetic and latex-allergic patients will be scheduled first on the surgical list. For diabetic patients, this reduces their starvation time and for the latex-allergic patients, it ensures clear air in the operating theatre.

6. Family history
   - Is there any family history of an adverse response to anaesthesia?
     - by asking this question, we are assessing the risk of malignant hyperthermia and suxamethonium apnoea (familial conditions that cause adverse reactions – see *Chapter 5*).

7. Social history
   - Does the patient smoke? How long have they smoked for?
     - advise to stop smoking 6–8 weeks prior to the surgical procedure; stopping smoking reduces complications related to airway reactivity and improves wound healing.
   - What is the patient's current alcohol intake?
   - Patient's functional status
   - Frailty score (using e.g. Clinical Frailty Scale).

2.2 A – Airway planning

A comprehensive airway assessment is vital for the safe conduct of anaesthesia.

The airway assessment helps to identify patients who may be difficult to intubate or bag–mask ventilate. Several bedside tests are used to help predict a difficult airway patient, but these do not have 100% accuracy.

Five key assessments are typically used to review a patient's airway:

1. Inspect the patient's face and neck for any obvious anatomical abnormalities or asymmetry.

2. Calculate the patient's Mallampati (MP) score.

This scoring system helps predict a difficult airway by establishing the view at the back of the mouth. The patient sits opposite the anaesthetist (at eye level) with their mouth open as wide as possible and tongue protruded.

■ Inspect the patient's oropharynx, looking at how easy it is to see their uvula and surrounding structures. *Figure 2.2* illustrates the scoring system for patients by the ease with which the anaesthetist can see the patient's uvula. The higher the MP viewing grade, the greater the probability of a difficult airway.

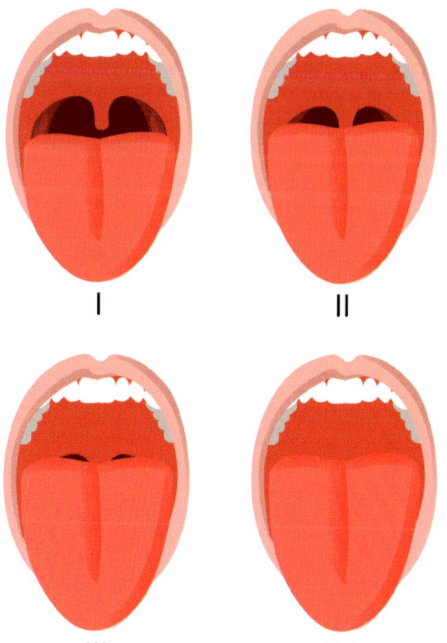

I II III IV

Figure 2.2: The ease with which a patient's uvula can be seen and their corresponding Mallampati score.
Class I: whole of uvula can be seen;
Class II: part of uvula;
Class III: only the soft palate;
Class IV: only the hard palate.

3. Ask the patient to open their mouth as wide as possible.

■ Measure the inter-incisor distance (i.e. the distance between the upper and lower incisors).
■ If the inter-incisor distance is less than three fingers' width (approximately 5 cm), this predicts that airway devices are going to be more difficult to insert. This is usually caused by temporomandibular joint (TMJ) problems.

4. Inspect the patient's teeth:

■ Dentition is important because airway instrumentation carries a risk of dental damage. Presence and location of dental work should be noted, along with any loose or damaged teeth. Buck or prominent teeth may be predictive of a difficult airway.

5. Determine the range of the patient's neck movements.

■ Ask the patient to extend and flex their head. Limitations in C1/C2 vertebral movement may be predictive of a difficult airway.
■ Assess a number of key anatomical distances:
  ● the **thyromental distance** (the distance between the thyroid cartilage and the patient's chin when the patient extends their head); a thyromental distance of <7 cm indicates there may be difficulty in inserting an airway device / maintaining ventilation (7 cm is roughly the width across four fingers when held together)
  ● the **sternomental distance** (the distance from the suprasternal notch to the chin, when the head is fully extended and the mouth closed); a sternomental distance of <13.5 cm is predictive of a difficult airway.

When assessing the patient's airway, it is important to note that none of the assessments is 100% accurate, but they act as a helpful guide.

2.3 B – Bloods and investigations

The preoperative assessment provides an opportunity to identify comorbidities that require further investigation or monitoring. The National Institute for Health and Care Excellence (NICE) published guidelines in 2016 on what preoperative investigations are indicated, depending on patient and surgical factors[2].

2.3.1 Patient fitness

To describe the patient's fitness prior to receiving anaesthesia, it is common practice to use the American Society of Anesthesiologists' (ASA) physical status classification. This descriptive scoring system based on the patient's comorbidities is used worldwide and follows criteria for selecting which grade a patient fits into.

There are six ASA classifications:

1. The patient is normal and healthy
2. The patient has a mild systemic disease (or is pregnant)
3. The patient has a severe systemic disease that limits their activity
4. The patient has a systemic disease which is a constant threat to their life
5. The patient is moribund and is not expected to survive without the operation
6. The patient is brain-dead, and their organs are being removed for the process of donation.

2.3.2 Surgical grade

The type of surgery is classified into a surgical grade[2]. *Table 2.1* shows the three different surgical grades (minor, intermediate and major (or complex)) and provides examples of each. This classification system is based on the invasiveness and length of the surgical procedure.

Table 2.1: Surgical grades

Surgical grade	Examples
Minor	Excising a skin lesion
	Draining a breast abscess
Intermediate	Primary repair of an inguinal hernia
	Excising varicose veins in the leg
	Tonsillectomy or adenotonsillectomy
	Knee arthroscopy

Surgical grade	Examples
Major (or complex)	Total abdominal hysterectomy
	Endoscopy resection of prostate
	Lumbar discectomy
	Thyroidectomy
	Total joint replacement
	Lung operation
	Colonic resection
	Radical neck dissection

Using the ASA classification and the surgical grades together can help determine which investigations are required preoperatively.

If the surgery is graded as 'minor', conduct the investigations shown in *Table 2.2*.

Table 2.2: Investigations to be made prior to minor surgery

Investigation	ASA grade		
	1	2	3 or 4
Full blood count (FBC)	No	No	No
Clotting profile	No	No	No
Kidney function	No	No	Only if patient is at risk of AKI*, i.e. increased age of the patient/nephrotoxins
Electrocardiogram (ECG)	No	No	Consider if there are no ECG results available for the past 12 months
Lung function tests/arterial blood gas	No	No	No

*Risk factors for acute kidney injury (AKI) include emergency surgery (especially if septic or hypovolaemic), intraperitoneal surgery, chronic kidney disease (if eGFR <60 ml/min/1.73 m²), diabetes, heart failure, age ≥65 years, liver disease, use of drugs with nephrotoxic potential in the perioperative period (e.g. NSAIDs).

FOR MINOR SURGERIES

In summary, for minor surgeries only conduct kidney function tests and an ECG in patients with an ASA grade of 3 or 4.

If the surgery is graded as 'intermediate', conduct the investigations shown in *Table 2.3*.

Table 2.3: Investigations to be made prior to surgery categorised as intermediate

Investigation	ASA grade		
	1	2	3 or 4
FBC	No	No	Consider for patients with cardiovascular or renal disease if symptoms have not been investigated recently
Clotting profile	No	No	Consider in patients with chronic liver disease
Kidney function	No	Only in patients at risk of AKI*	Yes
ECG	No	Only in patients with diabetes, cardiovascular disease or renal disease	Yes
Lung function tests / arterial blood gas	No	No	Seek advice from a senior anaesthetist

*Risk factors for AKI include emergency surgery (especially if septic or hypovolaemic), intraperitoneal surgery, CKD (if eGFR <60 ml/min/1.73 m^2), diabetes, heart failure, age $\geq$65 years, liver disease, use of drugs with nephrotoxic potential in the perioperative period (e.g. NSAIDs).

FOR INTERMEDIATE SURGERIES

In summary, for intermediate surgeries:
- ASA 1: conduct no tests
- ASA 2, 3 or 4: conduct a kidney function test and ECG
- ASA 3 or 4: conduct a full blood count, clotting profile (only in chronic liver failure), kidney function tests and lung function tests (if appropriate).

If the surgery is graded as 'major (or complex)', conduct the investigations shown in *Table 2.4*.

Table 2.4: Investigations to be made prior to surgery graded as major (or complex)

Investigation	ASA grade		
	1	2	3 or 4
FBC	Yes	Yes	Yes
Clotting profile	No	No	Consider in patients with chronic liver disease
Kidney function	Only in patients at risk of AKI*	Yes	Yes
ECG	In patients aged >65 years, who have no ECG results available for the past 12 months	Yes	Yes
Lung function tests / arterial blood gas	No	No	Seek advice from a senior anaesthetist

*Risk factors for AKI include emergency surgery (especially if septic or hypovolaemic), intraperitoneal surgery, CKD (if eGFR <60 ml/min/1.73 m^2), diabetes, heart failure, age ≥65 years, liver disease, use of drugs with nephrotoxic potential in the perioperative period (e.g. NSAIDs).

FOR MAJOR (OR COMPLEX) SURGERIES
In summary, for major (or complex) surgeries:
- ASA 1: conduct an FBC, kidney function (if AKI risk) and ECG (if >65 years)
- ASA 2: conduct an FBC, kidney function and ECG
- ASA 3/4: conduct an FBC, clotting profile (only if chronic liver failure), kidney function, ECG, and lung function tests (if appropriate).

2.3.3 Other investigations

In addition, there are some investigations that are not stratified by the patient's fitness and the surgical grade of their procedure. One way to remember these investigations is by the mnemonic **SHRUB**.

Swabs

Methicillin-resistant *Staphylococcus aureus* (MRSA) swabs are routinely taken, because MRSA-colonised patients will require decolonisation treatment before surgery. Swabs are taken from the nostrils and the groin.

At the time of writing, Covid-19 swabs are also required. However, this may change so please refer to current local guidance.

HbA1c

Take a blood test to measure the patient's HbA1c if they are diabetic and there is no HbA1c value available for the past 3 months. This provides an indication of their diabetic control and allows adjustment of their diabetic medications preoperatively (see *Section 2.4.1* on how diabetic medications are affected by the perioperative journey).

Radiation (an X-ray)

NICE does not recommend a routine chest X-ray prior to undergoing surgery. Cervical spine X-rays (extension and flexion views), to identify if a patient has conditions such as atlanto-axial subluxation (see *Key notes* box below), are indicated in the following conditions[2]:
- ankylosing spondylitis
- rheumatoid arthritis
- Marfan syndrome
- Down syndrome.

Urine dip

Conduct a urinary pregnancy test if the patient is of childbearing age, because GA and radiation exposure from intraoperative X-rays have implications for fetal development.

Blood products

Certain surgical operations have a higher risk of bleeding, and some patients have conditions that increase their bleeding risk. In both cases, these patients may require blood transfusions. A group and save ± a preoperative cross-match of packed red cells is required (see *Key notes* box below for more information). On occasion, clotting factor replacement or platelet transfusions

KEY NOTES

What is atlanto-axial subluxation and why do we worry so much about it?

Atlanto-axial subluxation is a condition where the C1 and C2 vertebrae are misaligned.

Patients with ankylosing spondylitis, rheumatoid arthritis, Marfan and Down syndrome are generally more at risk of developing atlanto-axial subluxation because their ligaments that hold the two vertebrae together are not as strong as normal. If the patient develops atlanto-axial subluxation, the consequences can be disastrous if the misaligned segments cause cord compression. Atlanto-axial subluxation can also occur traumatically if there is damage to the C1 or C2 vertebrae.

If atlanto-axial subluxation is present, we minimise movement of the patient's neck. Airway instrumentation may be conducted with video laryngoscopy, which reduces required neck movement.

KEY NOTES

Group and save and cross-matching

It is important to know the difference between conducting a group and save (G&S) blood test and cross-matching blood.

Group and save

A group and save blood test involves sampling the patient's blood in order to check their blood group and to assess if they have any abnormal antibodies. If blood is required, a cross-match can often be done from that sample and the units of blood issued. A G&S is often done when blood loss is unlikely but still a possibility.

Cross-match

Cross-matching blood is when the blood bank prepares blood products for us, and so you cannot do a cross-match without a G&S first!

The following types of blood products need a G&S and then a cross-match:

- Packed red cells
- Fresh frozen plasma
- Cryoprecipitate
- Platelets.

may be required preoperatively in order to minimise bleeding risks in patients with haemophilia or thrombocytopenia-related comorbidities.

It is not necessary to conduct a G&S and then cross-match blood for every patient undergoing a surgical procedure. NICE has provided us with guidelines as to when each of these tests is required (see *Table 2.5*)[2].

Table 2.5: The likelihood of a transfusion being required and the type of blood product that should be requested

Operative procedure	Chance of transfusion	Action required
Abdominal aortic aneurysm repair (elective)	Definite	Cross-match 4–6 units
Appendicectomy	Unlikely	G&S
Cystectomy	Definite	Cross-match 2 units
Hepatectomy	Definite	Cross-match 4–6 units
Hysterectomy (simple)	Unlikely	G&S
Lower segment caesarean section	Unlikely	G&S
Laparoscopic cholecystectomy	Unlikely	G&S
Oesophagectomy	Definite	Cross-match 4–6 units
Oophorectomy	Definite	Cross-match 4–6 units
Salpingectomy for ruptured ectopic	Likely	Cross-match 2 units
Thyroidectomy	Unlikely	G&S
Total gastrectomy	Definite	Cross-match 4–6 units
Total hip replacement	Unlikely	G&S

2.4 C – Comorbidities: medication management

Depending on surgical and patient factors, certain groups of regular medications need adjusting perioperatively.

2.4.1 Diabetic medications

Diabetic patients are at an increased risk of perioperative complications[3].

- Patients are required to fast prior to an operative procedure. As a result of this fasting and taking their usual diabetic medication, the patient's blood glucose may become erratic (with a risk of a patient having a hypoglycaemic episode).
- The 'surgical stress response' causes endocrine changes that affect cellular responses to insulin. This includes reduced sensitivity to insulin and increased cortisol levels, which stimulates gluconeogenesis.
- Diabetes is associated with immune system dysfunction, and so these patients are at an increased risk of developing postoperative infection and poor wound healing.

Due to these potential issues:

- All diabetic patients are to be first on the list for surgery
- Blood sugars monitored throughout the surgical procedure and pathway.

Table 2.6 demonstrates the common steps to be taken with different diabetic medications.

Table 2.6: Preoperative steps to be taken prior to surgery, depending on a patient's diabetic medication

Diabetic medication	Action to be taken
Oral hypoglycaemics	
Metformin	Omit lunchtime dose on day of surgery (regardless of whether the surgery is in the morning or afternoon)
SGLT-2 inhibitors	Omit all SGLT-2 inhibitors (including canagliflozin and dapagliflozin) 3 days prior to the operative procedure
Sulphonylurea	Omit sulphonylurea medications (including glibenclamide or gliclazide) on day of surgery

Subcutaneous hypoglycaemics	
Subcutaneous insulin	The night before surgery reduce subcutaneous (SC) basal insulin dose by one-third On morning of surgery do not administer the patient's usual morning insulin Prescribe patient an IV variable rate insulin infusion if this is required for prolonged surgery or difficult glycaemic control (this is also called a 'sliding scale'): ● The sliding scale contains 49.5 ml of normal saline with 50 units of Actrapid ● Alongside this, prescribe 5% dextrose or 0.9% saline as required by patient's blood glucose result ● Ward teams should check blood sugar values every 2 hours and alter the infusion according to patient's glucose result ● Stop the sliding scale when patient is eating and drinking, and return to their normal insulin regimen safely.

In general, oral diabetic medications can be restarted once the patient has returned to eating and drinking.

2.4.2 Steroids

Prescribe additional glucocorticoids to a patient taking >5 mg prednisolone per day or a patient known to have Addison's disease[4]. All of these patients are at risk of hypoadrenal crisis secondary to the surgical stress response.

In accordance with the Association of Anaesthetists, the Royal College of Physicians and the Society for Endocrinology, patients should receive:

■ hydrocortisone 100 mg IV at induction
■ followed by a continuous infusion of hydrocortisone at 200 mg IV over 24 h, until the patient can take double their usual oral glucocorticoid dose by mouth
■ this should then be tapered back to the appropriate maintenance dose, in most cases within 48 h, although this can be up to a week if the surgery is major/complicated.

Why do we require steroids for patients undergoing surgical procedures?

To understand the reason that we supplement steroids in patients with Addison's disease or with reduced steroid production, it is necessary to understand the hypothalamic–pituitary–adrenal (HPA) axis during a stress response (*Figure 2.3*).

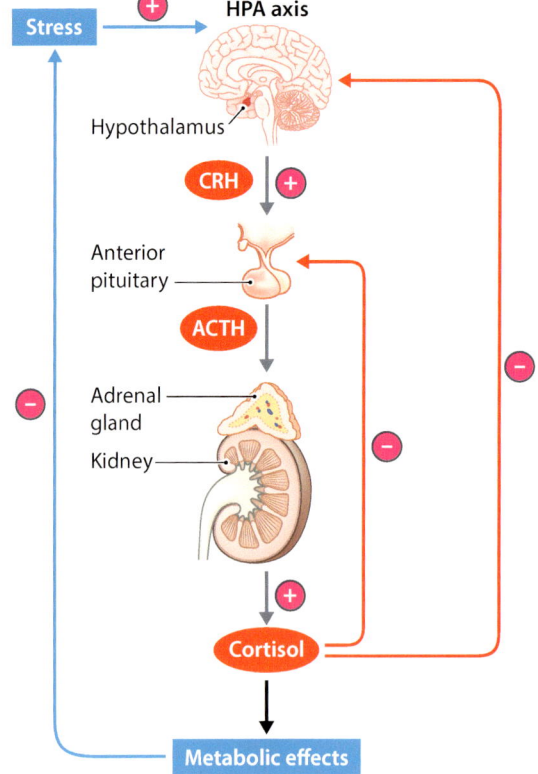

Figure 2.3: The HPA axis. Both exogenous steroid use and Addison's disease lead to reduced cortisol secretion from the adrenal glands.[5]

In periods of stress (which could be either psychological stress, illness/surgery or physical activity), the hypothalamus releases an increased level of cortisol-releasing hormone (CRH). This increases secretion of adrenocorticotrophic hormone (ACTH) from the pituitary gland, which has the net effect on the adrenal glands of increasing the levels of cortisol secretion. This cortisol plays a key role in glucose control, electrolyte maintenance and immune system regulation. Patients who have Addison's disease, or who have received long-term supplementary steroids, have an impaired ability to secrete cortisol from their adrenal glands. This means that in the postoperative period patients can experience an 'Addisonian crisis' or cardiovascular instability, with features including:

- malaise
- tiredness
- hypotension
- hyperkalaemia.

2.4.3 Anticoagulation and antiplatelet medications

Stopping anticoagulants and antiplatelet medications[6] preoperatively is dependent on the risk of thrombosis compared to the risk of haemorrhage, and so it is patient- and operation-dependent.

Warfarin

The management of warfarin depends on the patient's international normalised ratio (INR) (see *Table 2.7*).

Table 2.7: Management of warfarin preoperatively depending on the patient's INR

INR	Management
INR >1.5	Stop warfarin 5 days prior to procedure Reassess INR prior to surgery (the day before); if it is still raised (>1.5), prescribe 5–10 mg vitamin K
INR <1.5	Continue warfarin as normal. Reassess INR prior to surgery (the day before); if raised (>1.5), prescribe 5–10 mg vitamin K
Emergency when INR cannot be measured	Normalise INR with oral or IV vitamin K (5–10 mg) in repeated doses Prothrombin complex concentrate (Beriplex), which contains clotting factors II, VII, IX and X, can also be used (requires discussion with haematology)

After the surgical procedure, the patient should restart their warfarin, with daily INR checks to ensure they are in the correct INR range. While waiting for the INR to come into correct range, provide the patient with low molecular weight heparin (LMWH; normally enoxaparin 40 mg OD) to reduce their risk of developing a blood clot.

Aspirin and clopidogrel

Aspirin when taken at a dose of 75 mg OD is usually continued for elective surgery, because the antiplatelet effect is not enough to present a significant bleeding risk. However, clopidogrel is stopped 7 days prior to the surgery date.

In emergency situations where patients are taking antiplatelet agents it is advisable to seek haematological advice, because platelet administration may be required.

2.4.4 Oral contraceptive pill

If a patient is having major surgery, or a procedure that requires prolonged immobilisation of their lower limbs, they should stop taking their oral contraceptive pill (OCP)[7] 4 weeks before the operation date. This reduces their risk of developing a deep vein thrombosis (DVT) in the postoperative period.

If the patient would still like contraception during this time, transition them onto the progesterone-only pill. The OCP can then be restarted at the woman's first menses, 2 weeks after mobilising postoperatively.

2.4.5 Anti-epileptic and Parkinson's medications

All anti-epileptic and anti-parkinsonian medications must be continued perioperatively as there is a significant risk if they are stopped abruptly or missed. Patients should take their morning doses as normal with a small sip of water.

Convert oral doses to their IV equivalents if the patient will be starved for prolonged periods or will likely not tolerate oral medications postoperatively.

2.5 D – Drugs to provide

The most common medications to be administered preoperatively may be remembered as the **3 As**:

- **A**nalgesia
- **A**ntacids
- **A**nxiolytics.

2.5.1 Analgesia

Analgesia will be administered to the patient preoperatively, perioperatively and postoperatively.

This has been discussed in *Section 1.3*.

2.5.2 Antacids

Antacids are sometimes provided to patients who have an increased risk of aspiration on induction or waking. They increase the pH of the stomach contents, reducing the harm caused by aspiration, but they do not prevent aspiration from happening.

If the patient has gastro-oesophageal reflux disease (GORD), then they should take their prescribed medication. In some patient groups, e.g. obstetric patients undergoing caesarean section, routinely give antacids because they are at a higher risk of aspiration. The type of antacid provided is either ranitidine 150 mg or omeprazole 20 mg PO.

2.5.3 Anxiolytics

Anxiety before surgery is extremely common, but it doesn't usually prevent the surgery from taking place; calm reassurance from the theatre team is all that is required. There may be instances, however, such as with children, where this is not enough and medications are required.

Anxiolytics[8] typically include benzodiazepines such as temazepam PO or midazolam PO/IV.

2.6 D – DVT/VTE prophylaxis

After a surgical procedure, patients are at an increased risk of developing a deep vein thrombosis (DVT), which is when a thrombus (blood clot) forms in the deep veins of the body. For patients, a DVT can have a significant impact on their postoperative recovery, as they are associated with pain and reduced mobility, and require anticoagulation for at least 3 months.

KEY NOTES

Why are postoperative patients at a higher risk of developing a DVT?

To understand why postoperative patients are at an increased risk of developing a DVT, we must go back to Virchow's triad. Virchow's triad describes the three broad factors that are thought to contribute to a thrombus forming:

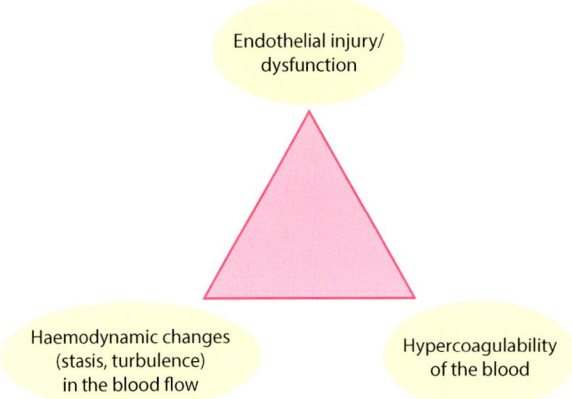

We must consider how each of these factors is affected by the surgical process:

1. Hypercoagulability

After a surgical procedure, the patient becomes hypercoagulable, with an increased tendency to form blood clots. Levels of tissue plasminogen activator (t-PA), which plays a key role in the formation of blood clots, increase after a surgical procedure.

2. Haemodynamic changes

As patients are relatively immobile in the postoperative period, blood pools in the venous system and this contributes to clots developing.

3. Endothelial injury/dysfunction

The invasive process of surgery causes damage to the endothelium of the venous system, and this increases the chance of clots forming.

Importantly, a DVT may progress to a pulmonary embolus (PE), which may cause:

- chest pain
- breathlessness
- hypoxia
- tachypnoea
- tachycardia
- cardiac arrest[9].

Correct risk assessment and prophylaxis to mitigate DVTs are an obligatory part of a hospital admission.

2.6.1 Risk assessment

NICE recommends that all surgical and trauma patients should be assessed to evaluate their venous thromboembolism (VTE) risk[10].

Broadly, the following surgical patients are at an increased risk of developing a VTE:

- Significantly reduced mobility for $\geq$3 days
- Hip or knee replacement
- Hip fracture
- Anaesthetic + surgical time being >90 minutes
- Surgery involving pelvis or lower limb with total anaesthetic time lasting >60 minutes
- Acute surgical admission with inflammatory or intra-abdominal condition
- Critical care admission
- Active cancer
- Age >60 years
- Dehydration
- Known thrombophilia
- Obesity
- Significant comorbidity, e.g. heart failure (HF), chronic obstructive pulmonary disease (COPD)
- Family history of VTE
- Use of hormone replacement therapy (HRT) or OCP
- Varicose veins with phlebitis
- Pregnancy or <6 weeks postpartum.

2.6.2 Methods of providing VTE prophylaxis

There are two types of VTE prophylaxis that are used: mechanical and pharmacological. The aims of these prophylactic measures are to counter the abnormalities in Virchow's triad that are seen in the postoperative period.

Mechanical prophylaxis

This aims to reduce the venous stasis that occurs in the postoperative period. It is initiated when the patient is admitted to hospital and stopped when the patient is mobile (which should be encouraged as soon as possible after surgery).

NICE recommends two different methods to provide mechanical prophylaxis:

1. Anti-embolism stockings (thigh or knee length)

These influence all three components of Virchow's triad. The stockings (see *Figure 2.4*) are made from elastic and reduce the risk of blood clots forming by gently compressing the patient's legs. This pressure prevents blood from pooling. Furthermore, the pressure from the stockings also improves endothelial wall function and is considered to enhance the breakdown of existing blood clots.

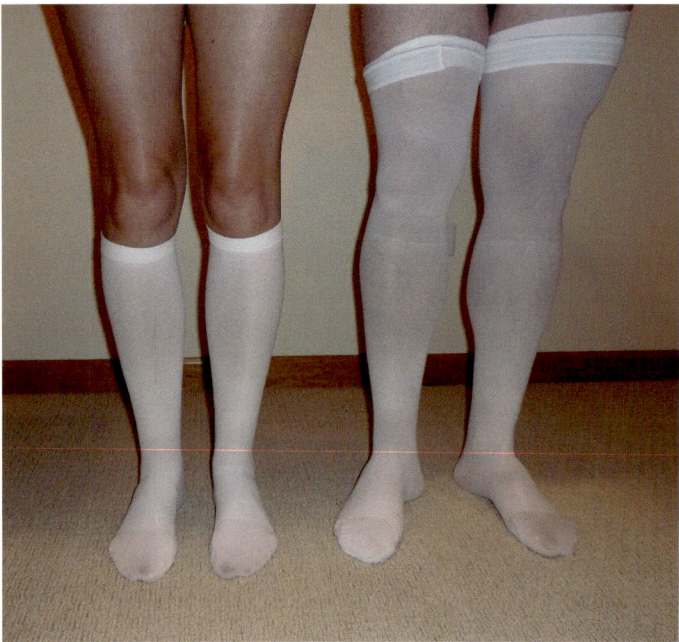

Figure 2.4: Knee-high and thigh-high versions of compression stockings to prevent DVT.

There are, however, contraindications to the use of anti-embolism stockings:

- Peripheral arterial disease
- Peripheral neuropathy
- Dermatitis, gangrene or a recent skin graft on the lower limb
- Severe leg oedema
- Limb deformity.

2. Intermittent pneumatic compression devices

These are air pumps with inflatable sleeves (see *Figure 2.5*). These sleeves cover the limb below the knee and go through a constant cycle of inflation and deflation, improving venous blood flow in the process. These are commonly used in the operating theatre and ICU alongside or instead of anti-embolism stockings.

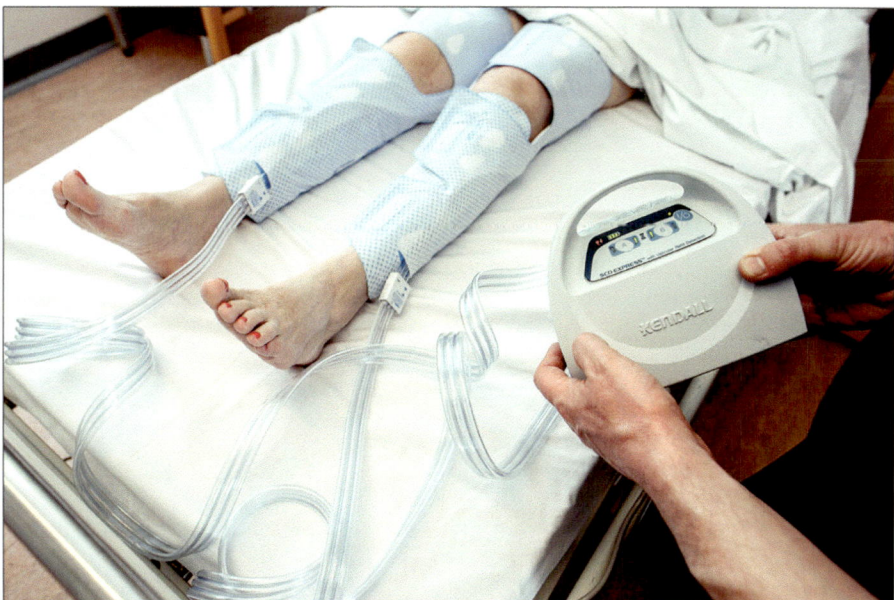

Figure 2.5: Application of intermittent pneumatic compression devices to both lower limbs.[11]

Pharmacological prophylaxis

Pharmacological prophylaxis 'thins' the blood by acting on the clotting cascade, and therefore reduces the risk of clot formation.

In general, all orthopaedic patients and other medium- or high-risk surgical patients should receive pharmacological prophylaxis, alongside mechanical prophylaxis against a DVT.

For all other patients, the choice is based on clinical risk assessment and judgement. NICE guidelines (NG89; 2018, updated 2019) state that the first-line medication for pharmaceutical prophylaxis should be enoxaparin (a LMWH). The usual prophylactic dose of enoxaparin is 40 mg SC OD; however, this dose is adjusted according to the patient's weight and renal function.

Postoperatively, NICE recommends maintaining the administration of enoxaparin for a period of time which depends on the surgical procedure undertaken and the patient's likely period of immobility (see *Table 2.8*).

Table 2.8: Choice and length of VTE prophylaxis

Procedure	Choice and length of VTE prophylaxis
Knee	Aspirin (75 mg) for 14 days or LMWH for 14 days, with anti-embolism stockings until discharge
Hip replacement	LMWH for 10 days, followed by aspirin (75 mg) for a further 28 days or LMWH for 28 days, combined with anti-embolism stockings until discharge
Thoracic surgery	Maintain LMWH for 7 days
Abdominal surgery	Maintain LMWH for 7 days (28 days if abdominal cancer resection)

It should be noted that patients who are already receiving anticoagulant medication (e.g. apixaban or warfarin) do not need to receive pharmaceutical prophylaxis because there will be no further reduction in their risk of DVT/VTE by providing both enoxaparin and their usual anticoagulant medication. However, if the patient is restarting warfarin, bridging with enoxaparin may be required as the patient is in a hypercoagulable state. Once the INR is in range, the enoxaparin should be stopped.

2.7 E – Entering surgical recovery

Patients undergoing major surgery, or those with significant comorbidities / complex care needs, require a higher level of nursing support. These individuals may require a high dependency or intensive care setting postoperatively.

Consider the appropriate destination of the patient by the level of care required:

Ward care: surgical ward care; patients will receive 1:8 nursing (i.e. 1 nurse to 8 patients).

Level 1 care: patients requiring more detailed observations or interventions (1:4).

Level 2 care: high dependency unit (HDU); patients will receive 1:2 nursing, with continuous monitoring.

Level 3 care: intensive care unit (ICU); patients will receive 1:1 nursing, with continuous monitoring.

2.8 F–Fasting

Patients undergoing GA should be appropriately fasted prior to the operation[12]. This decreases the risk of regurgitation and subsequent aspiration (see *Section 5.2* regarding aspiration). The rules for fasting, as described by the European Society of Anaesthesiology and Intensive Care (see bit.ly/ESAIC), are as follows:

Any patient having elective surgery, with no gastrointestinal comorbidities, should not:

- drink clear fluids for 2 hours preoperatively
- take solid food (including milk) for 6 hours preoperatively.

For children, avoid the following:

- formula milk, cow's milk or solids for 6 hours preoperatively
- breast milk for 4 hours preoperatively
- clear fluids for 2 hours preoperatively.

Fasting guidelines differ between hospital Trusts, and some elective surgery patients are now allowed to drink water up to 30 minutes before arriving in theatre.

2.9 Safety – conducting the WHO surgical checklist

The WHO introduced standardised checklists that could be used in any theatre across the globe, with the intention of improving team communication, increasing shared understanding and reducing errors. The WHO checklist begins with a team brief about the whole list at the start of the day, and each patient has an individual checklist with three distinct phases:

1. Before induction of anaesthesia (the 'sign-in')
2. Before the initial incision (the 'time out')
3. Before the patient leaves the operating theatre (the 'sign-out').

2.9.1 Prior to induction – sign-in

Prior to induction of anaesthesia the sign-in takes place; the patient provides confirmation of:

1. their identity (including full name, date of birth and address)
2. pertinent history, including when they last ate and their allergy status
3. the surgical procedure that is to be conducted
4. which side and site the operation will be (laterality).

The theatre team then confirms the following (remember these using the mnemonic **SHARP**):

- **S**ite of the surgery marked on the patient's body
- **H**aemorrhage risk (>500 ml blood loss)? If so, is the patient's blood group saved or cross-matched as required?
- Has the **A**naesthetic preoperative check been conducted?
- **R**isk of this patient having a difficult airway or aspirating their stomach contents?
- **P**ulse oximeter (and other appropriate/available monitoring) placed on the patient?

2.9.2 Before skin incision – time out

Before making the first incision into the patient's skin, conduct the 'time out' section of the WHO checklist (remember using the mnemonic **PAINS**):

- **P**rophylactic antibiotics given to the patient in the last 60 minutes?
- **A**naesthetic team addressed any patient-specific concerns that they have identified in their assessments?

- **I**maging for this procedure ready and visible to the required members of the team?
- **N**ursing team have ensured all the required surgical equipment for this procedure is present and appropriately sterilised?
- **S**urgical team have discussed the critical steps of this operation, the prospective operative duration, and the anticipated blood loss that the patient may undergo?

2.9.3 Before the patient leaves the operating room – sign-out

After the surgical procedure has finished and the patient is to be transferred to the recovery room, conduct the 'sign-out' section of the WHO checklist. As part of the sign-out, conduct the following checks:

- A count of all the instruments, swabs and needles that were used in the operative procedure, to ensure that they are all accounted for
- All specimens taken as part of the surgical process are labelled appropriately and sent to the lab
- A discussion is undertaken between the surgical, anaesthetic and nursing staff as to any specific factors that need to be managed for the patient postoperatively.

CHAPTER 3

Conducting anaesthesia

3.1	Induction of anaesthesia	49
	3.1.1 Rapid sequence induction	50
3.2	Maintenance anaesthesia	51
3.3	End of anaesthesia	53
	3.3.1 Enhanced recovery after surgery	53

We have previously discussed how the process of GA is divided into three distinct phases. Each of these phases represents differing activities that the anaesthetist will be conducting to transition the patient in and out of consciousness. These three phases are:

1. Induction of anaesthesia
2. Maintenance of anaesthesia
3. End of anaesthesia

Now that we have discussed the medications that are involved in providing a patient with GA, we will discuss what each of these stages of GA involves.

3.1 Induction of anaesthesia

Induction of anaesthesia is the first phase of providing GA. It describes the process of transitioning a patient from the awake state to an anaesthetised state. This phase of anaesthesia is routinely conducted using an intravenous/inhaled agent (see *Section 1.2*).

In clinical practice, the most commonly used drug is propofol (given IV). However, gaseous induction may be considered in the following circumstances:

- If the patient is a child. Gas induction in paediatric patients is relatively quick and less traumatic than attempting to get IV access. IV access is much easier to obtain once the child is unconscious (see *Figure 3.1*).
- IV access is difficult to obtain, e.g. small veins, highly needle-phobic patients or those with severe learning difficulties; gas induction may be a safer option and more tolerable for the patient.
- In some cases of difficult airways, gas induction does not reduce the upper airway tone as much as IV induction and it maintains spontaneous respiration. You can therefore prevent a difficult airway from becoming an impossible airway using this technique, e.g. epiglottitis requiring intubation.

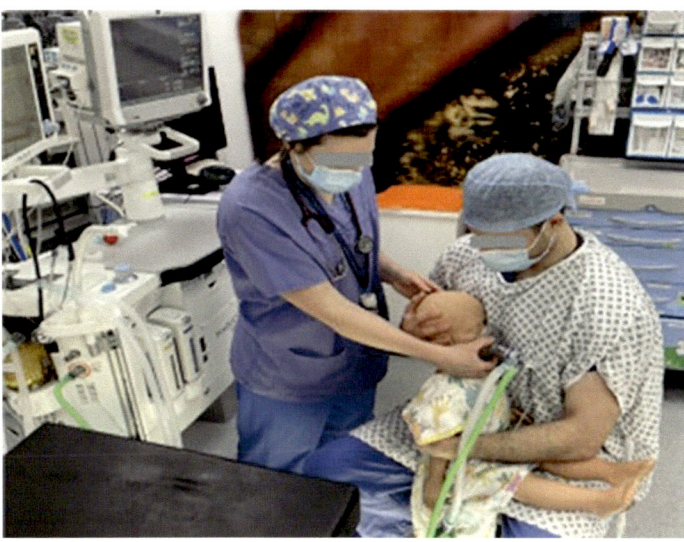

Figure 3.1: Gaseous induction of a child, using a mannequin[13].

3.1.1 Rapid sequence induction

Induction of GA, as described above, applies for fasted patients undergoing elective surgery. By fasting prior to the surgery, these patients have a reduced risk of aspirating their gastric contents.

In situations where a patient is not adequately starved, e.g. emergency surgery, the use of a rapid sequence induction (RSI) is required. As the name suggests, the induction of anaesthesia is 'rapid', using an induction agent and NMBD (if required) in 'sequence'. This results in intubating conditions within 30–45 seconds (almost 2 minutes quicker than standard intubation).

Indications for considering RSI include:

- patients who require emergency surgery and have not fasted for the appropriate amount of time
- patients who have an increased risk of gastric reflux, including:
  - those with conditions that cause delayed gastric emptying, e.g. autonomic gastroparesis secondary to diabetes or Parkinson's disease
  - all pregnant women who are in their second trimester onwards.

The process of conducting RSI is detailed below[14]:

1. Cannulate the patient and provide 100% O_2 for 3 minutes in order to ensure the patient is adequately pre-oxygenated. Give sleep-inducing dose of the GA agent and suxamethonium.
2. Apply cricoid pressure.
3. Attempt endotracheal (ET) tube intubation and confirm the correct position of the ET tube to ensure it is in the correct location (see *Section 4.3* for details on how to do this). Once the position of the ET tube is confirmed, release the cricoid pressure.
4. Provide ongoing anaesthesia (either an inhaled or IV GA agent).

KEY NOTES

What does cricoid pressure do to reduce the risk of aspiration?

In RSI, we apply pressure to the cricoid cartilage during anaesthetic induction (but before a neuromuscular blocker is provided). But how does this reduce the risk of the patient aspirating?

The upper oesophagus lies between the trachea and the cervical vertebrae. Pressure applied at the level of the cricoid cartilage occludes the upper oesophagus, preventing regurgitated contents from passing into the larynx and being subsequently aspirated into the lungs. The pressure is stopped when the ET tube is confirmed in its position (see *Section 4.3* for how we confirm the position of an ET tube).

3.2 Maintenance anaesthesia

Maintenance GA refers to the process of keeping the patient in an unconscious state. For most individuals, this involves providing a continuous supply of gaseous hypnotic agent. However, we can conduct maintenance GA using a continuous supply of the IV GA agent propofol. We call this form of maintenance GA total intravenous anaesthesia (TIVA).

To provide TIVA, the anaesthetist gives a controlled infusion of propofol and an opioid analgesic (typically remifentanil, which acts as an analgesic and further reduces the dose of GA agent required).

- ◼ TIVA is associated with a potentially increased risk of awareness during the operation. NICE recommends that patients receiving TIVA have bispectral EEG conducted perioperatively[15].
  - ● Bispectral EEG involves electrodes being placed on the patient's scalp to measure their brain activity (see *Figure 3.2*). By conducting bispectral EEG during maintenance anaesthesia, we can monitor a trend evaluation of depth of anaesthesia and alter agent doses to minimise side-effects and maintain anaesthesia more safely. An alteration in the trend representing a more awake patient can be evaluated and responded to quickly.

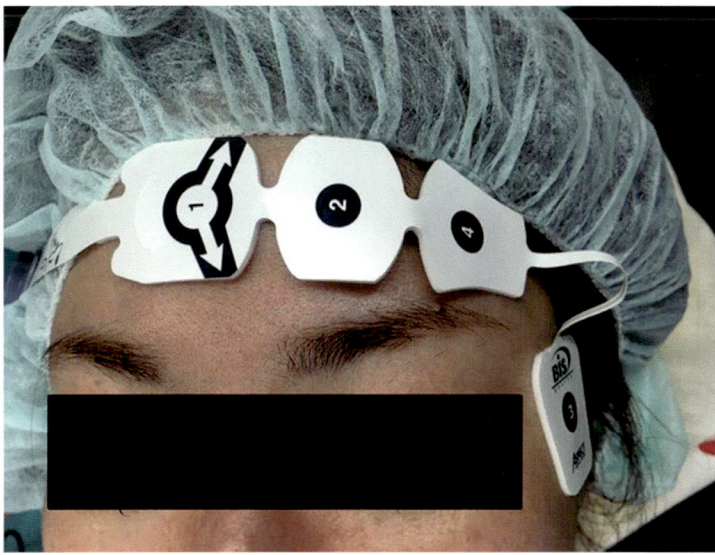

Figure 3.2: Bispectral EEG conducted with electrodes placed on the patient's scalp[16].

The indications for providing a patient with TIVA, instead of maintenance anaesthesia using gaseous hypnotic agents, include the following:

- If the patient is at risk of malignant hyperthermia. This is a genetic condition in which patients react to receiving gaseous hypnotic agents. See *Section 5.7* for more details on malignant hyperthermia.
- For patients that experience significant postoperative nausea and vomiting (PONV) with gaseous hypnotic agents, TIVA reduces the incidence of PONV.
- Inhaled anaesthetics prolong the QT interval. Therefore, in patients with a pre-existing prolonged QT, we avoid inhalation agents.

During both induction and maintenance GA, we monitor the patient to ensure the anaesthetic is effective and the patient is not having any complications.
This monitoring includes checking the following parameters:

- Inspecting the patient to see if they look comfortable
- Respiration rate
- Blood pressure (BP) (we monitor BP intra-arterially in long surgical procedures)
- Temperature
- Pulse oximetry
- Capnography (this is a measure of the amount of CO_2 being produced).

By monitoring these parameters, we can see whether the patient is receiving either too much or too little of the GA agent. An excessive administration of GA agent is expensive and leads to a greater risk of the patient experiencing adverse effects. If too little GA is provided, there is a risk of the patient becoming aware perioperatively. Features that indicate that the patient is not receiving enough GA include:

- Tachycardia and/or hypertension
- Movement of the patient
- Lacrimation
- Dilated pupils.

3.3 End of anaesthesia

When the surgical procedure comes to an end, we need to reverse the GA so that the patient can regain consciousness.

In order to do this, we conduct the following steps:

1. We stop providing the maintenance GA (either the inhalation or IV GA agent) and supply the patient with just 100% oxygen.
2. We reverse the patient's muscle paralysis using sugammadex (for non-depolarising agents).

Once the patient is respiring on their own, we can remove their airway device, so that they can breathe independently without an airway adjunct.

We then monitor the patient in recovery – when their observations are stable they can be transferred back to the ward.

3.3.1 Enhanced recovery after surgery

Enhanced recovery after surgery (ERAS) is a multidisciplinary approach that is designed to help patients recover quickly following surgery.

Under ERAS, teams are encouraged to assess and manage the parameters shown in *Figure 3.3* preoperatively, intraoperatively and postoperatively. Used together, these factors are known to significantly reduce the risk of complications and prolonged stay after surgery[17]. In terms of postoperative recovery the aims are:

- early return to fluids and oral intake
- to encourage mobilisation and physiotherapy for the patient
- management of the patient's pain (as discussed in *Section 2.5.1*).

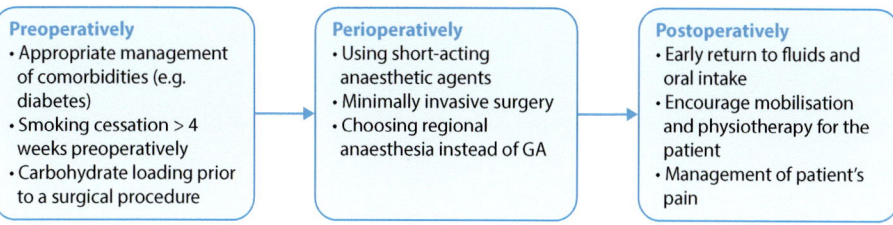

Figure 3.3: Factors identified within ERAS.

CHAPTER : 4

Airway management

4.1	**Airway adjuncts**	**57**
4.1.1	Oropharyngeal airway	58
4.1.2	Nasopharyngeal airway	59
4.2	**Supraglottic airway devices**	**62**
4.2.1	Laryngeal mask airway	62
4.2.2	i-gel airway device	64
4.3	**Subglottic airway devices**	**65**
4.3.1	Endotracheal tube	65
4.3.2	Tracheostomy and cricothyroidotomy	69

General anaesthesia reduces the airway tone and so, after induction, we require manoeuvres or devices to keep the upper airway open and allow ventilation to occur. The method of airway control and subsequent ventilation of the patient should be planned during the preoperative assessment.

The devices that we can use are classified anatomically:

- airway adjuncts – oropharyngeal/nasopharyngeal airways
- supraglottic (placed above the vocal cords)
- subglottic (placed below the vocal cords).

EXAM TIP

Learning these types of airways is important for your MCQs and your OSCE examinations. A common OSCE station involves the examiner asking you to talk through and demonstrate the insertion of each of these airway devices. Although you can only practise inserting these airway devices on mannequins and subsequently patients, we can provide you with the theoretical knowledge that underpins their use. Therefore, for each of these devices, learn the following key features:

- the type of airway device
- their method of insertion
- the indications for their insertion
- the common contraindications/complications.

4.1 Airway adjuncts

Airway adjuncts are found in theatre and on resuscitation trolleys. They are devices that can be inserted orally or nasally and are designed to sit within the naso-/oropharynx. They alleviate the obstruction caused by the tongue or soft palate when airway tone is reduced during GA (or if the patient is unconscious, e.g. in a cardiac arrest).

They are called 'adjuncts' because they aid airway patency when other manual airway manoeuvres have been performed, e.g. head tilt–chin lift or jaw thrust.

4.1

KEY NOTES

What is a head tilt–chin lift or a jaw thrust manoeuvre?

When a patient is in an unconscious state, there is a risk of their tongue falling backwards and occluding their oropharynx. When this occurs, the patient's airway becomes obstructed, preventing them from breathing adequately. It is heard as the sound of the patient snoring. Without intervention, the patient will have reduced ventilation, resulting in hypoxia and hypercapnia.

To prevent this from occurring, we use head tilt–chin lift and jaw thrust manoeuvres to maintain airway patency.

Head tilt–chin lift

This manoeuvre is conducted by tilting the patient's head backwards by applying pressure to their forehead and lifting the chin. This usually opens the airway (*Figure* 4.1).

The contraindication to this technique is a known/potential cervical spine injury or instability. If there is any C-spine concern, a jaw thrust manoeuvre is more appropriate (with in-line C-spine management).

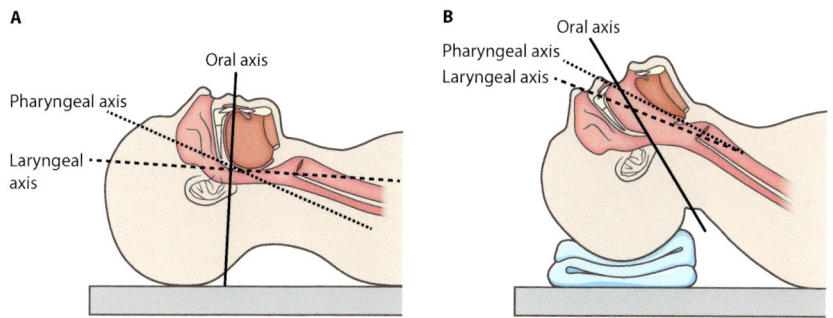

Figure 4.1: The head tilt–chin lift manoeuvre to open the airway. Part A shows head in normal position. In part B, a towel is placed behind the head, with the chin lifted upwards.

Jaw thrust

The clinician's index and middle fingers are placed behind the angle of the mandible and the jaw pushed anteriorly. Moving the mandible forwards lifts the tongue and can prevent it from occluding the airway (*Figure 4.2*).

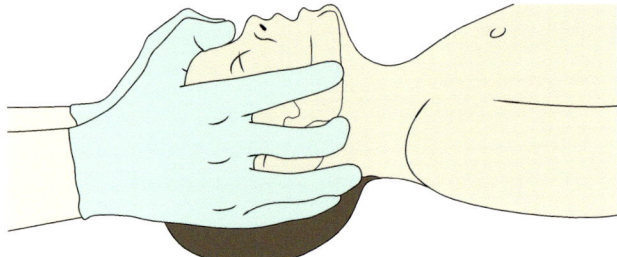

Figure 4.2: Opening the airway using the jaw thrust technique. The clinician's hands are placed behind the patient's mandibular heads, with the mandibular heads pushed upwards[18].

4.1.1 Oropharyngeal airway

Type of airway device

Oropharyngeal airways (OPAs) are also known as 'Guedel airways'. They are designed to maintain a patient's airway by preventing the tongue from falling backwards, causing airway occlusion.

They are curved to fit over the tongue and reach the oropharynx, with a flange that acts as a bite block and prevents the device migrating beyond the patient's teeth (see *Figure 4.3*). They allow ventilation through a hollow aperture in the middle.

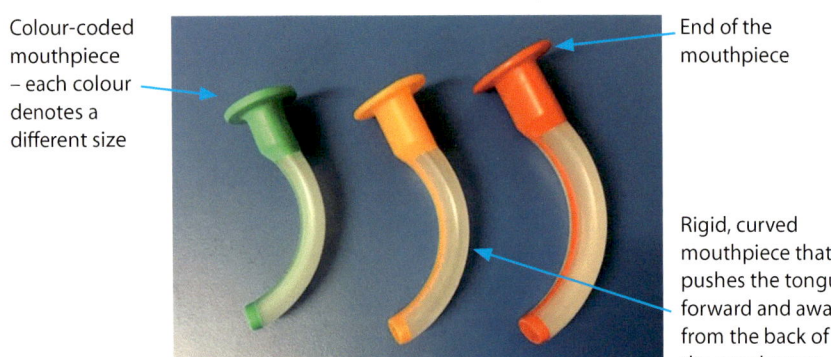

Colour-coded mouthpiece – each colour denotes a different size

End of the mouthpiece

Rigid, curved mouthpiece that pushes the tongue forward and away from the back of the oropharynx

Figure 4.3: Structure of an oropharyngeal airway device. Three different sizes are shown[19]. Green, size 2; orange, size 3; red, size 4.

Oropharyngeal airways are sized (see *Figure 4.4*) by measuring the device against the patient's face. With the tip at the angle of the jaw, the flange should align with the centre of the top teeth. Each device is colour-coded and sized by number.

Typical for an adult is the orange size, while the green may be used in teenagers. Smaller sizes are used in children.

Initially insert the oropharyngeal airway with the curved end pointed towards the palate of the mouth. As it is inserted, rotate it 180° gently so it curves over the tongue.

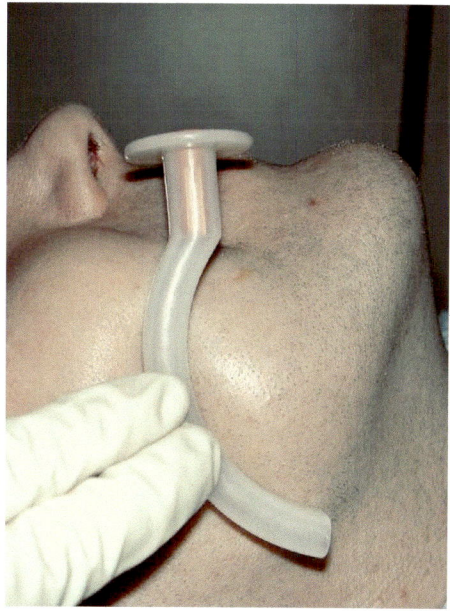

Figure 4.4: Sizing of an oropharyngeal airway device.

Indications for insertion

Insert an OPA for patients whose airway cannot be opened by a head tilt–chin lift and jaw thrust manoeuvre. OPAs tend to be used in emergencies or in theatre when the patient has obstructed prior to intubation.

Contraindications to and complications from inserting oropharyngeal airways

- Use with care in patients with oral trauma, because the insertion of the oropharyngeal airway device can lead to further oral trauma.
- They are poorly tolerated by patients who are semi-awake, as they induce the gag reflex. Nasopharyngeal airways are better tolerated in this context.

4.1.2 Nasopharyngeal airway

Type of airway device

The nasopharyngeal airway (NPA) provides a patent airway from the nose to the nasopharynx (see *Figure 4.5*). The distal end should sit beyond the base of the tongue.

Indications for insertion

- Much like oropharyngeal airways, nasopharyngeal airways are used for patients whose airway cannot be opened by a head tilt–chin lift and jaw thrust manoeuvre.

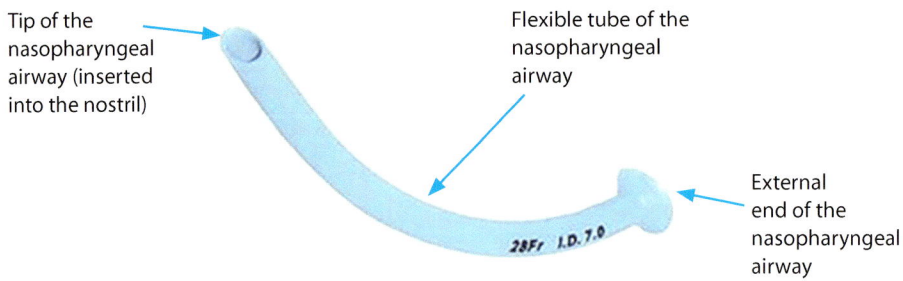

Tip of the nasopharyngeal airway (inserted into the nostril)

Flexible tube of the nasopharyngeal airway

External end of the nasopharyngeal airway

28Fr I.D.7.0

Figure 4.5: Key features of a nasopharyngeal airway device[20].

■ A nasopharyngeal airway can be used in patients for whom inserting an OPA would be contraindicated. It is usually better tolerated by patients and can stay in for longer.

Method of insertion

1. Nasopharyngeal airways must be sized appropriately to the patient: match the length of the nasopharyngeal airway to the distance between the patient's nose and their ear tragus (*Figure 4.6*).
2. Once measured, choose an appropriately sized airway device and cover it with lubricating gel.
3. Advance the device gently along the nasal passage. Generally, the right nostril is used because this makes the insertion easier (this is because of the natural curve of the NPA and how it fits along the nasal passage).

Contraindications to and complications from inserting a nasopharyngeal airway

The insertion of a nasopharyngeal device can cause trauma to the nasal passage. Complications can include:

■ epistaxis (nose bleeding)
■ damage to the base of the skull.

Inserting a nasopharyngeal airway is contraindicated in patients with facial injuries or with evidence of

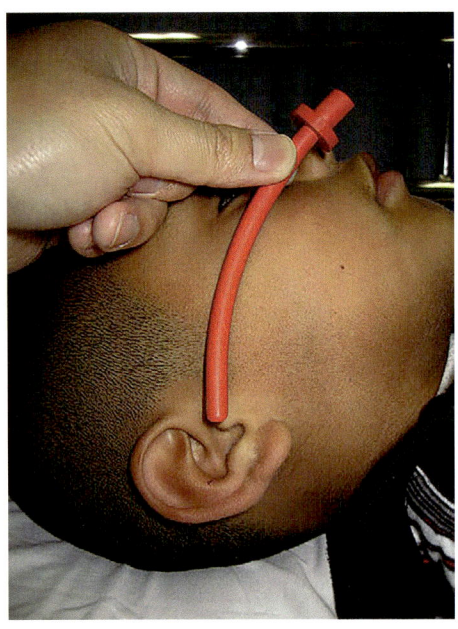

Figure 4.6: Measuring of the NPA[21].

basal skull fractures. Features of a patient having a basal skull fracture include (alongside a history of a head injury):

- the presence of darkened rings around the eyes (this sign is called raccoon eyes)
- bruising around the mastoid bone (Battle's sign)
- blood present at the tympanic membrane on otoscopy (known as a haemotympanum)
- cerebrospinal fluid (CSF) leaking from the ears (CSF otorrhoea) and ears (CSF rhinorrhoea).

4.2 Supraglottic airway devices

The 'glottis' is the opening between the vocal cords and so supraglottic devices sit above the glottis[22] (see *Figure 4.7*). Conversely, subglottic airway devices sit below the vocal cords.

There are two types of supraglottic airway device – the laryngeal mask airway and the i-gel.

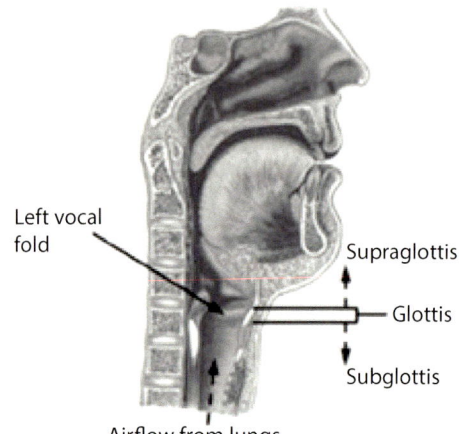

Figure 4.7: The position of the glottis. Airway devices that sit above this are termed supraglottic airway devices, and those that sit below are termed subglottic airway devices[23].

4.2.1 Laryngeal mask airway

The laryngeal mask airway (LMA) is a plastic tube attached to an elliptical mask with an inflatable cuff (see *Figure 4.8*). The mask is inserted into the patient's mouth so that it forms a seal around the patient's glottis (unlike ET tubes, that are placed past the glottis and into the trachea). The cuff is then inflated, forming an airtight seal. The positioning of the LMA is demonstrated in *Figure 4.9*.

Method of insertion

1. The patient is provided with 100% oxygen for 2–3 minutes, and induction of anaesthesia follows.
2. A jaw thrust manoeuvre will lift the tongue while the mouth is open.
3. Insert the tip of the LMA with the backplate against the palate, pushing gently until you meet

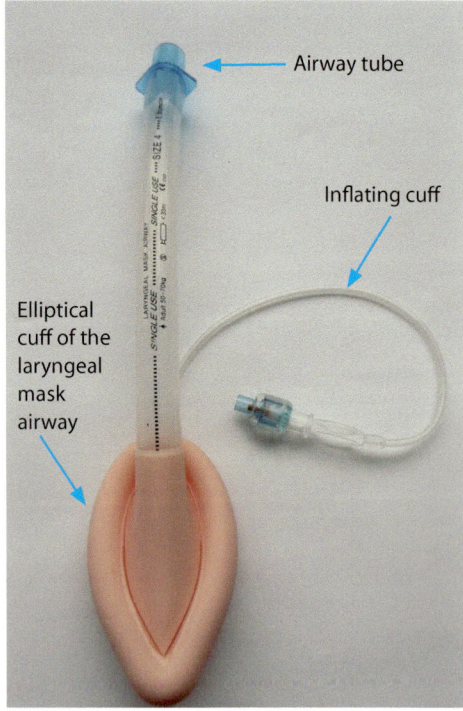

Figure 4.8: A laryngeal mask airway. The blue port on the right is for inflation of the cuff.

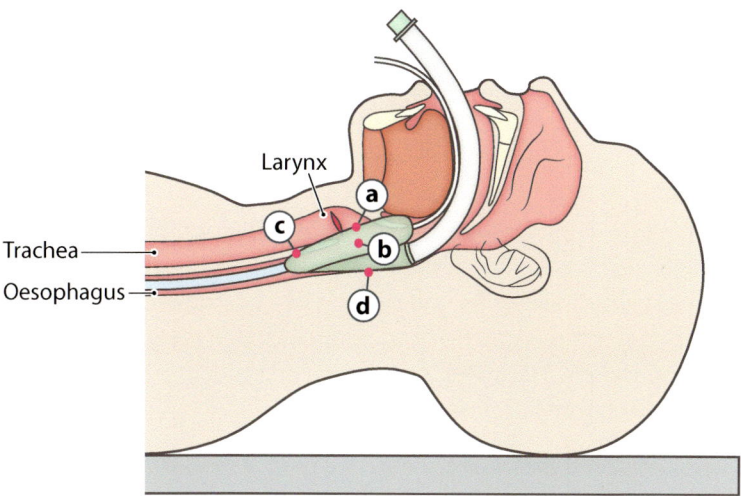

Figure 4.9: Positioning of the LMA after insertion. (a) anterior side of the LMA; (b) lateral side of the LMA; (c) tip of the LMA; (d) backplate of the LMA.

resistance (the cuff should be at the perimeter of the glottis, forming a seal once inflated).

4. The cuff is inflated to form a tight seal around the glottis.
5. Check the LMA is in the correct position and the patient is being adequately ventilated by looking at the capnography trace (this should demonstrate adequate CO_2 expiration), inspecting for chest expansion and auscultating the lung fields.

Benefits of using an LMA

1. The insertion of an LMA does not require laryngoscopy (as is required with an endotracheal intubation). Therefore, the technique for LMA insertion is easier to learn and a useful skill for any practitioner.
2. LMAs are on the resuscitation trolley alongside other airway devices as they are relatively easy to insert, meaning that advanced life support providers can use them without the presence of an anaesthetist.
3. They provide some protection from aspiration, whereas oro-/nasopharyngeal airways provide none.
4. LMAs can be used to rescue failed intubation (see *Section 4.3.2*).

Contraindications to and complications from using an LMA

- LMAs do not provide complete protection against aspiration.
- If not inserted properly, LMAs can cause oral mucosal damage.

4.2.2 i-gel airway device

The i-gel is a second generation supraglottic airway device (*Figure 4.10*) with a non-inflatable cuff, made from a soft, gel-like, thermoplastic elastomer. There are some differences in the preparation and insertion technique for i-gel® compared to an LMA.

   The non-inflatable i-gel cuff creates an anatomical seal around the pharyngeal, laryngeal and perilaryngeal structures. It incorporates a gastric channel (except size 1) which allows for the passing of a gastric tube to empty the stomach of fluid content; this gastric channel provides an early warning of regurgitation and may reduce its impact. An integral bite block also reduces the possibility of airway channel occlusion.

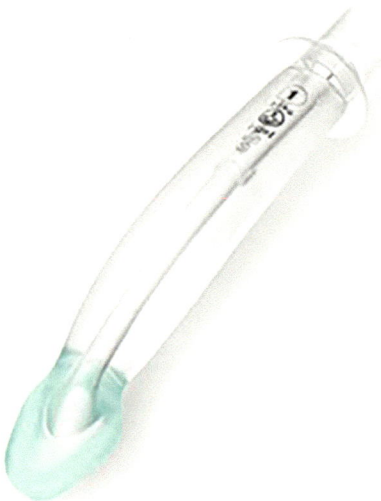

Figure 4.10: An i-gel airway device. The i-gel is a registered trademark of Intersurgical.

4.3 Subglottic airway devices

Subglottic airway devices may be placed through the mouth/nose or through the trachea (at the front of the neck).

There are two types of subglottic airway device:

1. Endotracheal tube
2. Tracheostomy and cricothyroidotomy

4.3.1 Endotracheal tube

An endotracheal (ET) tube is a hollow plastic tube that is inserted into the trachea, past the vocal cords. It has a balloon at the distal end that, when inflated, forms an airtight seal inside the trachea (see *Figure 4.11*). A laryngoscope is required to insert the ET tube – we will discuss what this is in the next section.

In adults, ET tubes are cuffed to protect against the risk of aspiration and to allow for effective ventilation. Paediatric ET tubes may be cuffed or uncuffed, depending on the patient's age. Young children have the narrowest point of their airway at the cricoid cartilage and pressure from an inflated cuff can cause mucosal injury and subsequent development of subglottic stenosis or oedema. In order to avoid post-extubation stridor (and failed extubation), an uncuffed tube may be used.

Note key features in the ET tube (*Figure 4.11*). The black lines are just proximal to the distal cuff. They should be placed at the level of the vocal cords. Centimetre markings are along the length of the tube, in order to secure the ET tube precisely and prevent movement, which might cause, for example, unilateral right main bronchus intubation. The typical depth of an ET tube is

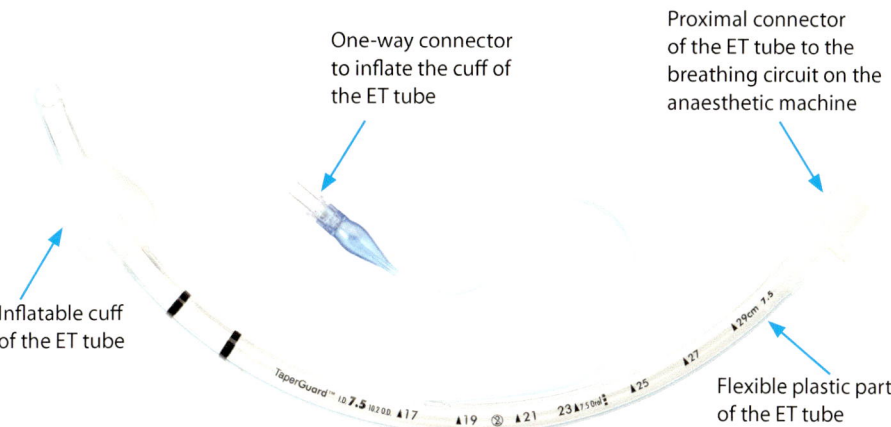

One-way connector to inflate the cuff of the ET tube

Proximal connector of the ET tube to the breathing circuit on the anaesthetic machine

Inflatable cuff of the ET tube

Flexible plastic part of the ET tube

Figure 4.11: Features of an ET tube (a standard, single-lumen ET tube as used in GA).

KEY NOTES

What is a bougie?

A bougie is a malleable plastic rod, with a flexible end, that is smaller in diameter and much longer than an ET tube. The bougie helps the anaesthetist intubate in individuals with very small or narrow airways. The bougie is inserted past the vocal cords and within the trachea, the ET tube can be 'slid' over the bougie and placed within the airway, allowing tracheal intubation to occur. This is possible because the bougie is thinner and more malleable, and acts as a stylet for ET tube placement. *Figure 4.12* demonstrates the bougie.

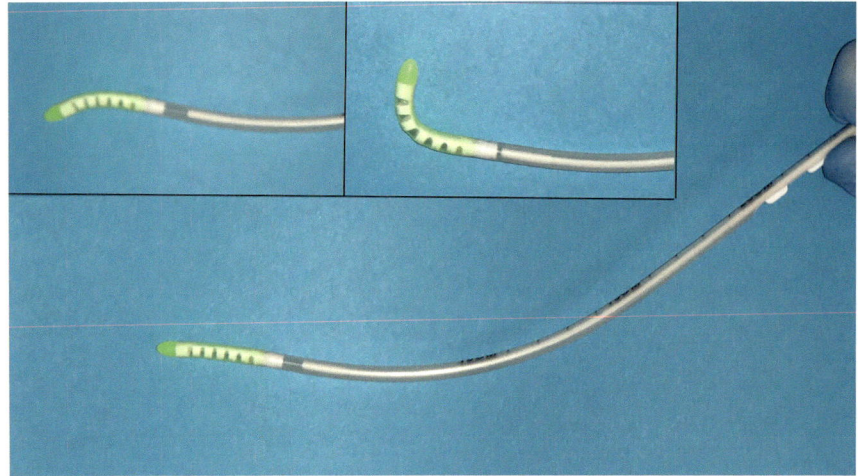

Figure 4.12: A bougie used for ET intubation. The bougie is a thin metal rod, with a curved end. It acts to 'guide' the ET tube into the correct position in individuals with a narrow throat[24].

23cm in men and 21cm in women – as shown by the centimetre markings on the tube.

The ET tube in *Figure 4.11* is a standard single-lumen ET tube used in GA. There are also nasal ET tubes, used mainly in maxillofacial procedures where oral surgical access is important, and double-lumen ET tubes used in thoracic surgery (because a double-lumen tube allows for the ventilation of one lung at a time if required).

What is a laryngoscope?

A laryngoscope is a device that is inserted into the mouth which allows the placement of the ET tube through the glottis.

There are a variety of different laryngoscopes available, and they have different pros and cons dependent on the context in which they are used.

The most commonly used laryngoscope is the Macintosh, which has a curved blade designed to fit into the oropharynx, and a small rounded tip which helps to lift the epiglottis. A light source at the end of the blade illuminates the laryngeal structures, allowing for direct visualisation and intubation. *Figure 4.13* shows the characteristic features of this device and *Figure 4.14* shows the anaesthetist's view when the laryngoscope is correctly placed. The blade tip is placed in the vallecula, and the epiglottis lifted to allow for passage of the ET tube through the glottis.

The ease of getting a view of the vocal cords with a laryngoscope can be anticipated in the airway section of a preoperative assessment. If the assessment indicates an anticipated difficult airway, or if the anaesthetist is finding it difficult to view the vocal cords during laryngoscopy (called

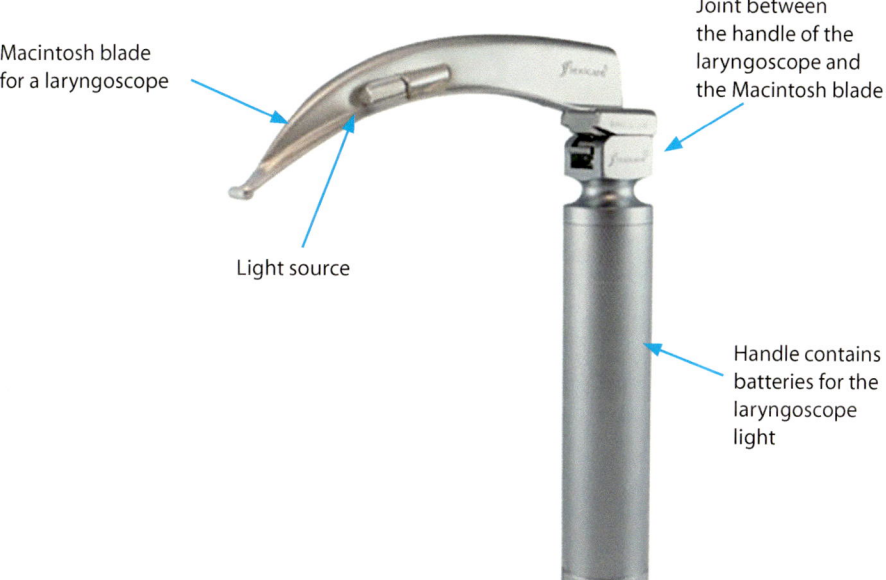

Joint between the handle of the laryngoscope and the Macintosh blade

Macintosh blade for a laryngoscope

Light source

Handle contains batteries for the laryngoscope light

Figure 4.13: A direct laryngoscope used to intubate patients with an ET tube. The laryngoscope is held in the left hand, with the right hand holding the mouth open[25].

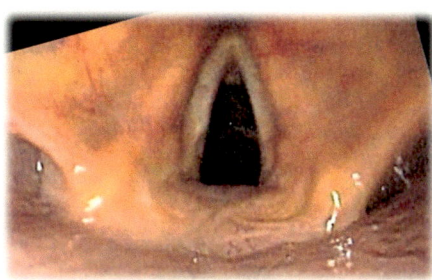

Figure 4.14: An anaesthetist's view of the vocal cords during tracheal intubation.

What is a video-assisted laryngoscope?

A video-assisted laryngoscope has an inbuilt video camera. Rather than the anaesthetist directly viewing the vocal cords, as shown in *Figure 4.14*, a real-time display on a screen (provided from a camera at the laryngoscope tip inside the oral cavity) is used to conduct intubation. This is useful for intubating difficult airways, because it allows indirect visualisation of the glottis opening with less movement of the cervical spine or mandible.

an unanticipated difficult airway), we may utilise a bougie or change our technique. If we change our technique, this may involve a different blade size or type, or alternative equipment such as a video laryngoscope.

Process of intubation

1. The patient is provided with 100% oxygen for 2–3 minutes and induction of anaesthesia follows. We call this period of oxygen delivery **pre-oxygenation**.
2. With the patient supine, the laryngoscope is inserted into the right side of the patient's mouth. It is advanced, gently pushing the tongue to the left side until the blade tip reaches the vallecula. The laryngoscope is then lifted upwards and away to elevate the larynx and allow visualisation of the tracheal inlet.
3. The ET tube is inserted through the vocal cords until the black lines on the ET tube are about to disappear from view.
4. Inflate the cuff of the ET tube to form an airtight seal (*Figure 4.15*).

Confirming the correct placement of an ET tube is paramount – check five key things (remember these using the mnemonic **CASTE**):

- **C**apnography trace should have started and identified that the patient is producing carbon dioxide consistently.
- **A**uscultate both lungs, listening for equal air entry bilaterally and that there are **S**ymmetrical chest movements. Check specifically for symmetry in the lung movements because the tube may have moved / be placed into one of the bronchi (this is usually the right bronchi as it's straighter than the left and therefore, easier for the tube to migrate into).
- Check for the presence of **T**ube misting. Condensation in the ET tube provides confidence that air from the lungs is moving through the ET tube.
- Finally, auscultate the **E**pigastric region, listening for stomach gurgling and observing for abdominal distension. The presence of either of these signs indicates that the tube may have been placed in the oesophagus. Note unidentified oesophageal intubation is life-threatening.

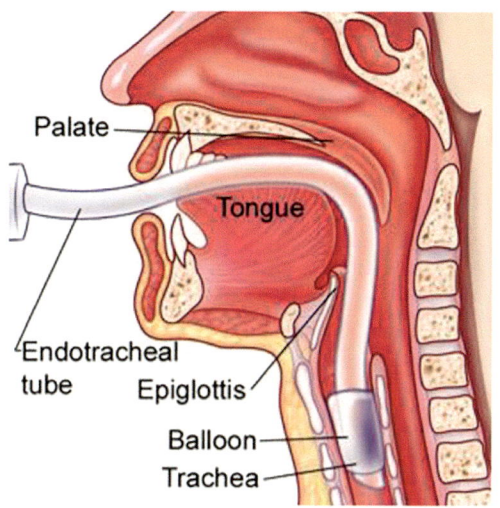

Palate

Tongue

Endotracheal
tube

Epiglottis

Balloon

Trachea

Figure 4.15: Position of ET tube after tracheal intubation[26].

If the anaesthetist is unsure that the ET tube is in the correct position, they should always remove it and reattempt tracheal intubation whilst maintaining oxygenation. This is because incorrect intubation can have disastrous consequences. Accidental intubation of the oesophagus will cause the patient to become hypoxic and desaturate, which is ultimately fatal. Intubation of one bronchus can cause barotrauma/volutrauma of the lungs.

Complications from insertion

- Insertion of the laryngoscope blade risks trauma to structures within the mouth and oropharynx. Dental damage, sore throat and hoarseness may occur.
- As previously discussed, accidental endobronchial or oesophageal intubation can occur if the ET tube is misplaced. This should be identified quickly using the checks detailed above.

4.3.2 Tracheostomy and cricothyroidotomy

Tracheostomy and cricothyroidotomy are subglottic airway procedures. A tracheostomy tube is inserted between the first and second tracheal rings, while a cricothyroidotomy inserts an airway through the cricothyroid membrane of the larynx. In general cricothyroidotomies are done in an emergency (as they are quick to conduct), while tracheostomies are planned, and used for prolonged ventilation.

Indications for a tracheostomy

There are three main indications:

1. Longer-term mechanical ventilation – a tracheostomy in ICU is usually performed for this reason
2. Facilitating weaning from mechanical ventilation
3. Upper airway obstruction, e.g. in ENT/maxillofacial oncology resections.

The insertion of a tracheostomy device is a routinely performed procedure on ICU. This is because a tracheostomy is less stimulating of laryngeal reflexes, such as cough and gag, than an ET tube, and facilitates mechanical ventilation without high doses of sedatives.

Complications of a tracheostomy

Early complications:

- The hole that forms the tracheostomy can become blocked with secretions or blood clots
- Displacement of the tracheostomy tube, or placement of the tube within a false passage
- Pneumothorax from insertion.

Late complications:

- Stenosis – long-term tracheostomies are associated with subglottic stenosis (narrowing of the airway below the epiglottis). This complication has been reported in up to 2% of all patients receiving a tracheostomy.

Indications for a cricothyroidotomy

The single indication for its performance is in an emergency where all other methods of oxygenation have failed and emergency airway access is required in order to save life.

Difficult airways

Previous sections have discussed airway assessment and how it helps to predict potentially difficult airway management. In the context of ET intubation, the patient may require repositioning and the passing of a bougie. If this is not possible, alternative methods of oxygenation and anaesthesia need to be considered. When oxygenation is not possible, it is necessary to consider a tracheostomy/cricothyroidotomy procedure.

When the preoperative assessment indicates potential difficulty, multiple plans are made with extra anaesthetists and extra equipment, in order to ensure safe anaesthesia and airway management. This may include video laryngoscopy and awake/asleep fibreoptic endoscopic intubation[27].

The Difficult Airway Society has created guidelines[28] for oxygenation in the context of an *unanticipated* difficult airway (see *Figure 4.16*). As per the

KEY NOTES

Emergency front of neck access

Emergency front of neck access (FONA) involves securing the patient's airway via the anterior aspect of the neck to provide emergency alveolar oxygenation. This includes cricothyroidotomy and tracheostomy. It forms the very last, life-saving stage in airway management when other techniques have failed to establish a patent airway. Indications for FONA include situations when attempts to manage the airway through other techniques have failed, or urgent situations with high-risk airways. This includes patients with upper airway obstruction from head and neck tumours, traumatic injuries to the face and neck, and severe airway oedema secondary to burns or anaphylaxis.

guideline, if intubation attempts have failed (up to three attempts allowed), insertion of a supraglottic airway device, e.g. laryngeal mask airway (LMA), is the next step. If this fails, bag–mask ventilation (when a ventilation bag, with a mask, is placed over the nose and mouth) is commenced in order to wake the patient.

If neither intubation nor ventilation is possible (can't intubate, can't oxygenate – CICO), cricothyroidotomy will be required and will be life-saving.

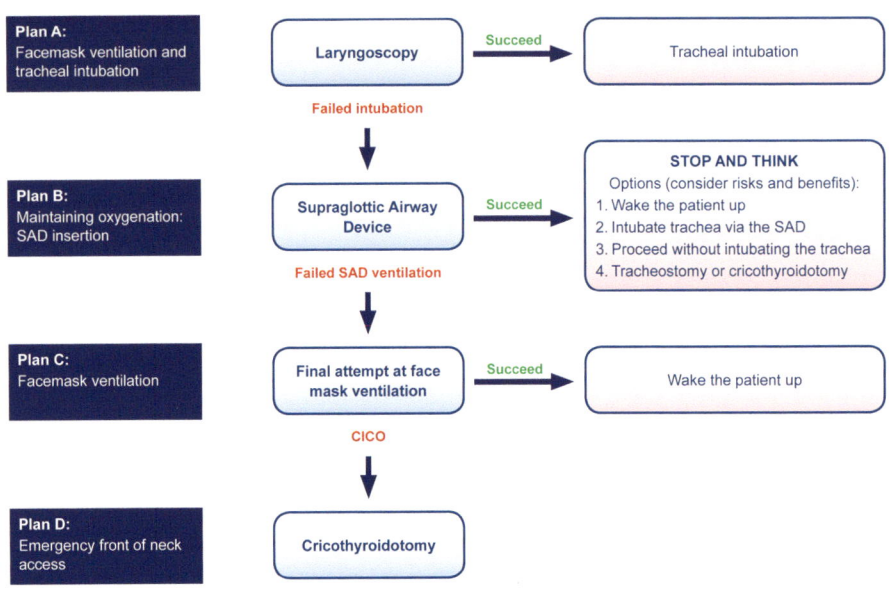

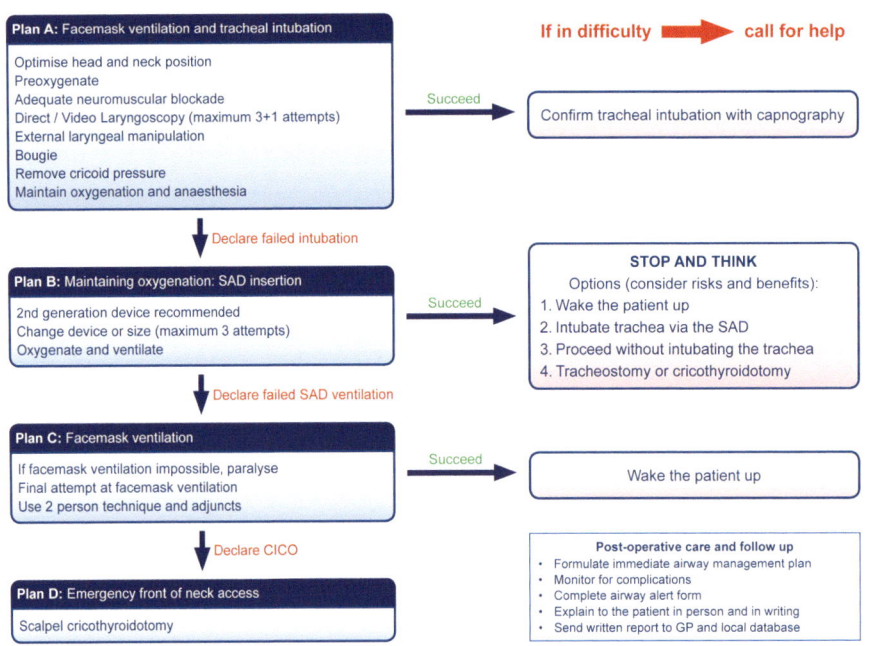

Figure 4.16: Difficult Airway Society guidelines[28] for the management of unanticipated difficult intubation in adults.

CHAPTER 5

Complications in anaesthesia

5.1	Anaphylaxis	74
5.2	Aspiration of gastric contents during anaesthesia	75
5.3	Atelectasis	77
5.4	Awareness during general anaesthesia	79
5.5	Bronchospasm	80
5.6	Laryngospasm	82
5.7	Malignant hyperthermia	84
5.8	Suxamethonium apnoea (pseudocholinesterase deficiency)	85
5.9	Shivering ± hypothermia	86

There are many complications that can be associated with anaesthesia. In this chapter we have listed the most common complications and how to appropriately manage these.

5.1 Anaphylaxis

Anaphylaxis[35] is a severe allergic reaction to a trigger and can be life-threatening. Sometimes patients are aware of the allergen that triggers anaphylaxis, but this may not always be the case.

The clinical features of an anaphylactic reaction include:

- hypotension, reactive tachycardia
- cutaneous flushing
- rash or urticaria
- angioedema (swelling of the skin and mucous membranes), resulting in hoarse voice and difficulty swallowing
- wheeze.

When conducting GA, there can be multiple potential allergens, and recent research has quantified the risk in the UK as 1:12 000 anaesthetics[29]. Listed below are the common triggers for anaphylaxis that have been recorded:

- Muscle relaxants (the causative agent in 60% of GA anaphylaxis cases)
- Latex allergy (the causative agent in 20% of GA anaphylaxis cases)
- Antibiotics (the causative agent in 15% of GA anaphylaxis cases).

Due to the severe and life-threatening nature of anaphylaxis, when any patient develops unexplained hypotension and/or bronchospasm during anaesthesia, it is appropriate to consider anaphylaxis as a potential cause.

Management

When anaphylaxis is suspected, prompt and immediate management is required. The most concerning feature in an awake patient is the presence of angioedema of the face or airway. If angioedema presents in the tongue and laryngeal mucous membrane areas, the swelling can occlude the patient's throat, leading to the loss of their airway and an inability to breathe.

1. Remove any potential triggers (if possible) that could be causing anaphylaxis (e.g. latex gloves, antibiotics being infused).
2. Provide the patient with 100% oxygen via a non-rebreathe mask.
3. Administer adrenaline (0.5 mg IM). Repeat this dose of adrenaline if there are no improvements in the patient's symptoms after 5 minutes (up to two doses).
4. Administer a 500 ml fluid bolus of 0.9% saline (chlorphenamine 10 mg IV and hydrocortisone 100 mg IV may be given, but are no longer included in the ALS guidelines).
5. To confirm an anaphylactic reaction, take a blood test for mast cell tryptase quantification at the time of the reaction, at 1–2 hours after the reaction and 24 hours later.

5.2 Aspiration of gastric contents during anaesthesia

Patients are fasted prior to receiving GA to reduce their risk of aspirating gastric contents perioperatively[30]. If there are concerns over the extent of a patient's fasting or whether the patient is at an increased risk of aspirating, conducting an RSI is one option because this reduces the chance of aspiration.

An aspiration event is defined as the inhalation of gastric contents into the respiratory tract. The aspirated content typically enters the right main bronchus (because the right bronchus is straighter than the left bronchus) and settles within the lungs.

Risk factors for aspirating gastric contents perioperatively can be remembered using the mnemonic **SAIDS**:

S – the type of **S**urgery the patient is undergoing
- Patients undergoing abdominal surgery and laparoscopy are at an increased risk of regurgitating and aspirating their gastric contents.
- This is because, during these operative procedures, increased intra-abdominal pressure will affect the gastro-oesophageal sphincter pressure gradient and may increase the likelihood of gastric contents entering the oesophagus and pharynx.

A – **A**naesthetic factors associated with the surgery
- As discussed in *Chapter 4*, the use of a non-definitive airway device increases the risk of aspiration (if regurgitation occurs) because they are not protective.

I – patients with an **I**ncompetent lower oesophageal sphincter
- Patients with a history of GORD or a hiatus hernia are at an increased risk of regurgitating their gastric contents.

D – the presence of **D**elayed gastric emptying
- Patients with delayed gastric emptying are more likely to have food contents still present in their gastrointestinal (GI) system after the standard 6-hour fasting time.

S – a patient with a full **S**tomach (patient is unfasted)
- In an emergency case, if the patient has not fasted for the appropriate amount of time, then the risk of regurgitation is increased; these unfasted patients require an RSI if anaesthesia cannot be delayed.

Presentation

If an aspiration event occurs, then patients may develop symptoms of respiratory irritation (pneumonitis) perioperatively. These symptoms and signs include coughing, tachypnoea and difficulty in ventilation.

The suspicion that a patient may have aspirated during a surgical procedure is always taken very seriously. If aspiration occurs, there is a risk of airway obstruction that may lead to impairment of ventilation and hypoxia, as well as aspiration pneumonia or pneumonitis (inflammation due to stomach acid).

Management

If aspiration occurs or is suspected, then conduct the following steps:

1. Thorough suction of the airway to remove gastric contents. Note that direct laryngoscopy may be required to visualise the airway.
2. The airway device that is *in situ* may need exchanging, e.g. the patient has an LMA inserted, and a definitive airway is required for ongoing management.
3. A chest X-ray may be required (to assess if aspirated contents have gone into the lungs).
4. Bronchoscopy and lavage are performed if there is heavy soiling of the bronchial tree or there is evidence of respiratory compromise.

5.3 Atelectasis

Atelectasis[31] is a condition that is caused by alveolar collapse. There are multiple proposed mechanisms as to how this collapse occurs; two are described below:

Compression atelectasis

Compression atelectasis occurs if the abdominal contents compress the lungs when the patient lies supine, and this reduces air entry into the basal lung areas.

Absorption atelectasis

If the patient is being ventilated perioperatively, they are initially provided with 100% oxygen, which differs from the composition of normal room air (78% nitrogen and 21% oxygen). When inhaling normal room air, nitrogen usually remains in the alveoli (thereby inflating the alveoli) and oxygen diffuses across the alveolar membrane and into the bloodstream. However, if the patient is receiving 100% oxygen, then more oxygen will diffuse across the alveolar membrane and into the bloodstream, reducing the volume of gas present within the alveoli. This results in the relative collapse of the alveoli, causing atelectasis.

Presentation

Clinically significant atelectasis typically presents within the first 24 hours after surgery with the following symptoms and signs:

- ongoing oxygen requirement (unexpected)
- bi-basal quiet/absent breath sounds
- desaturation on exertion.

Risk factors for developing postoperative atelectasis include:

- GA
- pre-existing lung pathologies (e.g. COPD, asthma, bronchiectasis)
- positive pressure ventilation (PPV) – this is a type of ventilation used for patients when they receive GA to ensure oxygen delivery and removal of carbon dioxide
- intra-abdominal surgery
- obesity.

Investigations

The best investigation to determine the presence of atelectasis is a chest X-ray. Features on a chest X-ray that indicate the presence of atelectasis include (see *Figure 5.1*):

- lung or lobar collapse (in very severe cases)
- hemi-diaphragm elevation on the side of the atelectasis.

Management

If a patient develops atelectasis in the postoperative period, provide them with chest physiotherapy and appropriate analgesia (this predominantly involves deep breathing exercises). The physiotherapy attempts to re-inflate the collapsed section of lung (incentive spirometry).

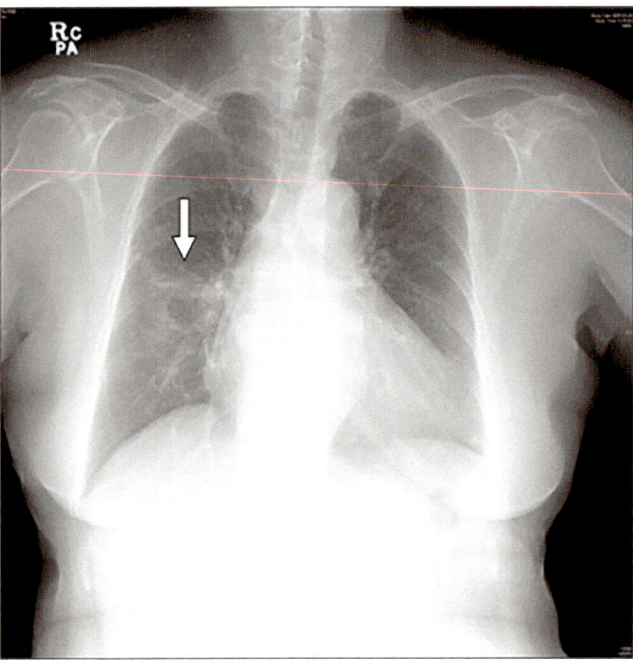

Figure 5.1: Chest X-ray of an individual with atelectasis and collapse of the right middle lobe[32].

5.4 Awareness during general anaesthesia

Awareness during GA[33, 34] may occur at any stage from induction to emergence. It occurs in roughly 1 in 19000 general anaesthetics. It can be divided into two types:

1. explicit awareness, which defines conscious awareness and recall of events
2. implicit awareness, which defines perception without conscious awareness.

Avoidance of awareness is a priority for an anaesthetist because it will clearly be extremely distressing and may have prolonged adverse psychological effects on patients. There are several risk factors for awareness under GA:

- Equipment failure
- Use of muscle relaxants
- Inadequate anaesthetic dose (inadvertent)
- Patient factors such as age, metabolism, concurrent use of drugs such as amphetamines.

Management

It is advised that if a patient can recollect part of their surgical procedure, the medical team should take the following steps:

1. Apologise to the patient, express regret and take their concerns seriously.
2. Provide a structured interview and questionnaire to detail what specific features of their perioperative episode they can remember.
3. Refer the patient for psychological support.
4. Explore potential reasons as to how this awareness could have occurred and discuss future events for the patient (i.e. how to make sure that this does not occur again).

5.5 Bronchospasm

Bronchospasm[35] occurs when the bronchial smooth muscle contracts, causing constriction of the bronchial tree. This reduces air entry to the alveoli, making the patient breathless (tachypnoeic) and wheezy.

The risk of bronchospasm occurring perioperatively is 0.2%. However, this risk is higher if the patient has a known respiratory pathology, such as asthma or COPD (where the incidence rises to 2%).

Risk factors for developing bronchospasm include:

- any instrumentation of the lower airway
- history of smoking
- history of atopy
- recent upper respiratory tract infection (URTI)
- respiratory pathology (e.g. asthma, COPD).

Presentation

- An **expiratory** wheeze on lung auscultation or audibly along the breathing circuit.
- The expiration phase of the patient's breathing will be prolonged.
- Capnography will show a characteristic 'shark-fin appearance' (*Figure 5.2*). This is not diagnostic of bronchospasm, but indicates that there is airway obstruction (a wider time differential of carbon dioxide release from different alveoli, leading to a gradient in the trace).

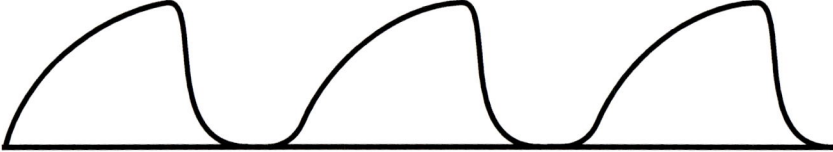

Figure 5.2: Characteristic 'shark-fin' capnography trace seen in patients with bronchospasm.

Management

If you suspect bronchospasm, provide 100% oxygen.

Bronchospasm is a feature of anaphylaxis and if signs and symptoms point towards anaphylaxis, then treat accordingly (adrenaline administration in this instance should resolve the bronchospasm).

Bronchospasm in isolation should respond to the following treatment:

1. Increasing the dose of inhaled anaesthetic agent induces bronchodilatation, but be aware that increasing the anaesthetic may reduce the patient's blood pressure.
2. Check the airway device. The device may have become dislodged and be stimulating structures to induce bronchospasm, e.g. the ET tube has moved distally and is touching the carina. Simply repositioning the device may resolve this.
3. If the bronchospasm has not resolved, nebulised salbutamol (2.5 mg) will promote further bronchodilatation (IV salbutamol can also be considered).
4. Consider the use of magnesium sulphate / theophylline / ketamine if bronchospasm is ongoing or worsening.

5.6 Laryngospasm

Laryngospasm[36] is a reflex where the larynx constricts, and this results in the partial or complete closure of the patient's vocal cords. It is a commonly occurring complication, affecting around 1% of patients undergoing GA. It should be managed quickly because delayed treatment can result in severe hypoxia and death.

Presentation

The presentation of laryngospasm depends on the extent of the closure of the vocal cords.

- If the vocal cords are partially shut, the patient will develop an **inspiratory** stridor perioperatively.
- If the cords are completely closed, the patient will have absolute obstruction of their airway, which will result in rapid and profound hypoxia as oxygen delivery is impossible. Although effective management of laryngospasm can be performed in a few simple steps, this is a clinical emergency.

Risk factors

There are several potential causes of laryngospasm which can be divided into anaesthetic, patient and surgical factors.

- Anaesthetic factors
  - insufficient depth of anaesthesia
  - irritation to the larynx or glottis by mucus or blood
  - airway manipulation causing laryngeal or glottic stimulation.
- Patient factors
  - younger age
  - airway hyper-reactivity: patients with asthma, COPD or a concurrent upper respiratory tract infection are at an increased risk of developing laryngospasm
  - current tobacco smokers.
- Surgical factors
  - surgery on the thyroid gland or on the oesophagus can damage or interfere with surrounding nerves, and this increases the risk of laryngospasm
  - surgery in and around the airway (e.g. a tonsillectomy) has a risk of introducing foreign material (usually blood and clots) around the vocal cords that may induce laryngospasm – the material can be hidden behind the uvula.

Management

First, attempt to identify the potential cause of the patient's laryngospasm, promptly remove this trigger and give the patient 100% oxygen.

Management of laryngospasm involves application of positive end-expiratory pressure initially.

If these measures fail then a bolus of IV anaesthetic agent, e.g. propofol, may be sufficient.

Then consider a rapid-acting muscle relaxant (e.g. suxamethonium) in addition to the IV anaesthetic agent. If a GA agent and NMBD have been given to resolve laryngospasm it is prudent to intubate the patient and attempt extubation in a controlled environment and without time pressure.

5.7 Malignant hyperthermia

Malignant hyperthermia[37] is an autosomal dominant condition that is triggered in certain individuals after administration of inhaled GA agents or suxamethonium.

The condition affects 1 in ~50000 patients who receive GA and the mortality rate from the condition is approximately 5%.

The pathophysiology of malignant hyperthermia is unknown. It is considered that susceptible patients have abnormalities in the sarcoplasmic reticulum of their skeletal muscle (specifically, in the ryanodine receptor) which is responsible for 80% of cases. As a result, exposure to either inhaled GA agents or depolarising muscle relaxants leads to an increased calcium concentration in the skeletal muscle cells during the acute phase of the condition.

Presentation

The presentation of malignant hyperthermia differs in the early and late stages. Initially there is:

- increased CO_2 production seen on capnography and hypoxia (increased oxygen requirement)
- increased muscle rigidity (specifically masseter spasm)
- cardiac arrhythmias including sinus tachycardia, supraventricular or ventricular arrhythmias.

In the later stages of the condition, the patient can experience a rapid increase in body temperature to above 38.8°C. Following such a temperature rise, signs and symptoms of cardiovascular instability, metabolic acidosis and rhabdomyolysis occur.

Treatment

Malignant hyperthermia mimics other conditions in its initial presentation, but if the condition is *suspected* then prompt treatment is required:

1. Get help and stop the precipitating agent.
2. Flush the anaesthetic machine with 100% O_2 and actively cool the patient.
3. Maintain anaesthesia with an IV agent (propofol is ideal) and a ventilation circuit free from inhaled GA agents.
4. Administer dantrolene: starting dose 2.5 mg/kg with 1 mg/kg boluses up to 10 mg/kg maximum.
5. Treatment of hyperkalaemia/acidosis/arrhythmia/AKI as required.
6. Discuss with ICU regarding further treatment and halt the surgical procedure safely.

5.8 Suxamethonium apnoea (pseudocholinesterase deficiency)

Suxamethonium apnoea[38] is a rare complication observed in patients who receive suxamethonium muscle relaxant. Patients with this condition have an abnormality in the enzyme acetylcholinesterase (AChE), which plays a key role in the breakdown of ACh. The deficiency in this enzyme leads to a prolonged effect of the suxamethonium, leading to prolonged paralysis.

The abnormality in AChE can be inherited in an autosomal recessive manner and it is particularly common amongst Persian Jewish communities. However, the condition can also be acquired in the following states:

- Pregnancy
- Liver/renal failure
- Carcinomatosis.

Presentation

The presence of suxamethonium apnoea may be suspected intraoperatively when the paralysing effects of suxamethonium don't wear off in the expected time period. If suxamethonium apnoea has not been suspected and anaesthesia ceases, then the patient will make no respiratory effort, but signs of awareness may become apparent, e.g. tachycardia, hypertension, lacrimation.

Treatment

It is essential to maintain or restart anaesthesia once suxamethonium apnoea is suspected. The patient will likely require transfer to intensive care because there is no reversal for suxamethonium, and the effects may last up to 24h.

Monitor the patient's muscle contraction ability by using a peripheral NMJ monitor and assessing the patient's response. Once the patient has recovered and regained muscle use, test the patient's peripheral cholinesterase activity (through a blood test) to help confirm the diagnosis.

5.9 Shivering ± hypothermia

Shivering[39] is common in the postoperative period, occurring in 20–70% of patients who receive GA. Overall, postoperative patients are at an increased risk of hypothermia due to anaesthesia-induced thermoregulatory impairment and having been exposed to a cold environment in the operating theatre.

Not all shivering is related to a fall in core body temperature; it is also a consequence of the experience of anaesthesia, surgery and pain.

Severe postoperative shivering is less common and more concerning because it increases oxygen consumption, resulting in hypoxaemia and a raised lactic acid.

Treatment

The treatment of hypothermia involves providing patients with warmed blankets, air heaters and warm IV fluids to increase the core body temperature. Shivering is usually self-limiting.

CHAPTER 6

Local anaesthesia

6.1	What is local anaesthesia?	88
6.2	Types of local anaesthesia	89
6.3	Complications of local anaesthesia	91

6.1 What is local anaesthesia?

A local anaesthetic is so called because it achieves loss of sensation only in the area in which it is administered.

Local anaesthetic drugs belong to two distinct chemical groups, esters (e.g. tetracaine) and amides (e.g. lidocaine and bupivacaine), but they generally all have the suffix '-caine'.

Drugs in the ester group are shorter-acting and have a higher potential for adverse side-effects, therefore most local anaesthetics in clinical use are amides.

Examples of areas of application for localised anaesthesia:

6.1

- topically to numb the skin for IV cannulation or procedures involving the eye
- peripheral nerves in the gums for single dental extractions
- skin layers for suturing of a wound.

This is in contrast to regional anaesthesia (see *Chapter 7*), which has the following as examples of areas of application:

- peripheral nerves to block whole body regions/parts
- fascial planes to achieve spread across several nerves using one injection
- around the spinal cord to achieve anaesthesia at a particular spinal cord level or the nerve roots as they leave the spinal cord in the epidural space.

Method of action

All local anaesthetics achieve their effect by diffusing across the cell membrane of nerves and binding to the voltage-gated sodium channels on the inside of the cell wall. In doing this, nerve conduction is prevented, and motor/sensory signals are not transmitted along the nerves that contain local anaesthetic.

- Sensory nerves that carry pain signals are smaller than other nerves and are readily blocked by local anaesthetic.
- Motor nerves are larger and require higher concentrations of local anaesthetic agent.

There are many different types of amide local anaesthetic, all with different properties that relate to their chemical structure. Lidocaine and bupivacaine are two of the most common ones.

6.2 Types of local anaesthesia

Lidocaine

Formula: $C_{14}H_{22}N_2O$

General information: lidocaine is the most common and widely used of all the local anaesthetic agents in general medical practice.

It sometimes comes mixed with adrenaline. The adrenaline promotes vasoconstriction at the site of application, reducing the absorption of the local anaesthetic agent and increasing its concentration, prolonging its action and allowing a larger dose to be used, usually for a wider area.

Adrenaline is contraindicated when administering local anaesthesia to peripheral anatomical structures with a single or unpredictable blood supply, because the adrenaline may cause vasoconstriction that leads to ischaemia. Be aware that lidocaine, like all local anaesthetics, comes as a 1% or 2% solution (see box below for explanation on this), so you must always check carefully which one you want!

Features:
- **Uses**: can be applied topically (e.g. throat spray to numb the throat) or by superficial injection (commonly used for suturing).
- **Onset of action**: local anaesthesia is provided within 1–5 minutes of application.
- **Duration**: with adrenaline 90 minutes, and without adrenaline 30–60 minutes.
- **Maximum dose**: max. dose for an adult is 3 mg/kg (7 mg/kg when mixed with adrenaline).

EXAM TIP

What does 1% mean?

The concentration of the local anaesthetic agent can be written either as a percentage or in mg/ml and this can make things confusing when we are trying to consider the amount of drug a patient requires. However, it is important for your MCQs that you know how the conversion from percentage to mg/ml works. A common question you may be asked is to calculate the maximum amount of local anaesthetic in millilitres (ml) that you can administer to a patient who is, say, 60 kg.

Drug concentrations that are written as percentages can be thought of as drug quantity in milligrams per millilitre (mg/ml). A 1% solution contains 10 mg/ml, and a 0.5% solution contains 5 mg/ml for any compound. From this, we can work out the maximum amount in millilitres of a certain percentage of solution that we can provide to a patient, in one administration.

The maximum dose of lidocaine we can give (with no adrenaline) is 3 mg/kg, so for a 60 kg patient, that is equivalent to a maximum of 180 mg. 1% lidocaine has 10 mg/ml, so we can give up to 18 ml of 1% lidocaine.

Bupivacaine

Formula: $C_{18}H_{28}N_2O$

General information: bupivacaine is a longer-acting local anaesthetic agent compared to lidocaine.

Features:

- **Uses**: superficial injection (commonly used after a surgical incision for postoperative pain relief) or regional anaesthesia (see *Chapter 7*).
- **Onset of action**: bupivacaine has a slower onset of action than lidocaine, with anaesthesia occurring in 6–10 minutes from application.
- **Duration**: 2–3 hours.
- **Maximum dose**: max. dose in adults of 2–2.5 mg/kg (2.5–3 mg/kg when mixed with adrenaline).

6.3 Complications of local anaesthesia

There are several complications that can arise from the administration of local anaesthetic agents.

Persistence of local anaesthesia symptoms

Local anaesthetic injection around nerves has the potential to damage the nerve, either by direct trauma of the needle or by injection of the local anaesthetic directly inside the nerve, as opposed to around the nerve.

Regional anaesthetic techniques (see *Chapter 7*) are more likely to damage important nerve structures, because the technique involves depositing local anaesthetic around large nerves; for example, a spinal anaesthetic deposits local anaesthesia directly around the spinal cord. The deficit is usually temporary, resolving within 12 weeks.

Allergic reactions

Allergic reactions to the local anaesthetic agents are rare. Any reaction could also be due to the preservatives mixed within the local anaesthetic.

Anaesthetic toxicity (overdose)

Infiltration anaesthesia involves the administration of a local anaesthetic agent into the subcutaneous tissue. However, if there is inadvertent injection of this anaesthetic agent into the arterial or venous system, then the patient can develop systemic adverse effects (bradycardia, hypotension, etc.).

Presentation of local anaesthetic overdose

Local anaesthetics are not selective to sodium channels within nerves and so, if inadvertently injected into the systemic circulation, the local anaesthetic will bind to sodium channels in the brain and heart. If the dose is injected intravascularly then local anaesthetic toxicity may occur. Characteristic features of local anaesthetic toxicity include:

- peri-oral tingling
- anxiety/confusion
- hypotension, cardiac arrhythmia, cardiac arrest
- tinnitus, tremors, twitchiness
- seizures.

These features typically occur within 5–10 minutes of the local anaesthetic injection.

Management of local anaesthetic overdose

1. Stop local anaesthetic administration.
2. Call for help.
3. A–E assessment including 100% O_2 administration and airway support as required.
4. Intralipid – 20% lipid emulsion (administered IV) given at 1.5 ml/kg then 15 ml/kg/h infusion.

CHAPTER 7

Regional anaesthesia

7.1	**Peripheral nerve blocks**	**95**
7.1.1	Types of peripheral nerve block	96
7.2	**Neuraxial anaesthesia**	**98**
7.3	**Epidural anaesthesia**	**99**
7.3.1	Clinical uses of epidural anaesthesia	99
7.3.2	Complications of epidural anaesthesia	100
7.4	**Spinal anaesthesia**	**104**
7.4.1	Complications of spinal anaesthesia	105

Regional anaesthesia describes a group of techniques that block specific nerves that supply discrete regions of the body.

Regional anaesthesia can be used as the sole technique or in combination with GA. The approach depends on surgical factors:

- For isolated digital/hand surgery, a regional technique is a commonly chosen option.
- In longer body compartment surgery, a regional technique may not be appropriate; blocking one set of nerves would not be sufficient to prevent the pain sensation of surgery.

Regional anaesthesia is associated with faster recovery and a reduced number of adverse effects (compared to GA), including reduced PONV. Regional anaesthesia can be classified as:

- peripheral nerve blocks (i.e. blocking nerves away from the spinal cord)
- neuraxial techniques (which involve blocking nerves at or immediately surrounding the spinal cord) – this includes spinal anaesthesia and epidural anaesthesia.

7.1 Peripheral nerve blocks

Peripheral nerve blocks target specific nerves or groups of nerves anywhere along their course. The technique usually targets the nerve itself or fascial planes through which the nerves traverse. The effects of the resulting 'block' are evident from the site of injection and distally, so if the ulnar nerve is blocked at the elbow, the ulnar distribution beyond the point of injection will be anaesthetised. The nerve block procedure requires[40]:

- sound anatomical knowledge of peripheral nerves
- knowledge and understanding of the use of ultrasound to find the nerves to block
- knowledge of equipment, e.g. needle length required, use of ultrasound scan (USS) guidance (*Figure 7.1*).

a

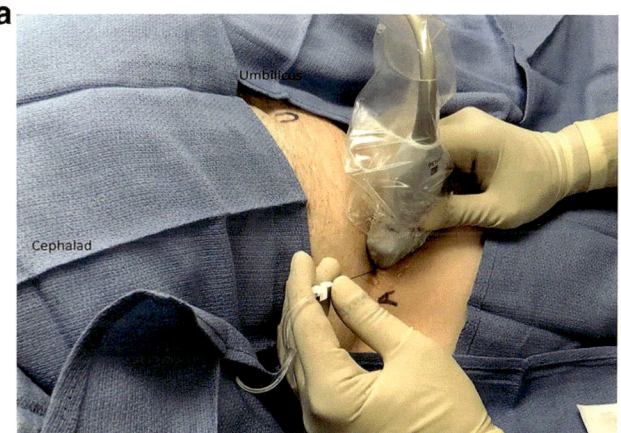

b

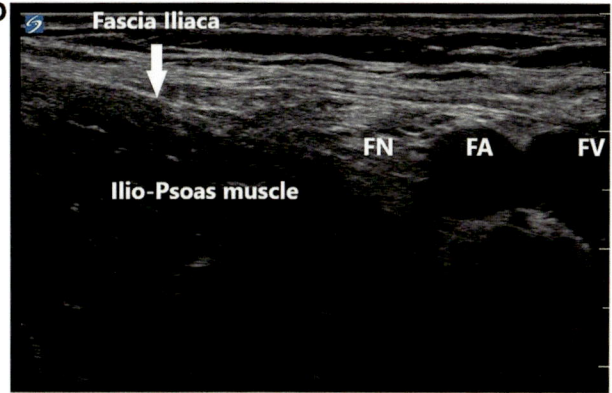

Figure 7.1: (a) Infra-inguinal fascia iliaca block and femoral nerve block; note the probe position at the inguinal crease and approach of the needle from lateral to medial. (b) ultrasound image at the inguinal crease showing the fascia iliaca, femoral nerve (FN), femoral artery (FA), femoral vein (FV), and iliopsoas muscle[41].

Uses

1. To provide regional anaesthesia to an area of the body, with or without the need for a GA.
2. In combination with GA, where the main aim is to provide analgesia perioperatively as part of a multimodal analgesia plan.

Contraindications to administering a peripheral nerve block

- Absolute contraindications
  - patient refusal
  - allergy to local anaesthetic
  - infection at the site of injection.
- Relative contraindications
  - coagulopathy
  - movement disorders
  - pre-existing neuropathy.

7.1.1 Types of peripheral nerve block

Depending on the anatomical site of injection, regional anaesthesia may block single nerves, groups of nerves or a whole nerve plexus, as shown in *Figure 7.2*.

Complications

Complications that can arise from conducting a peripheral nerve block can include:

- iatrogenic nerve injury (a direct nerve injury by the needle)
- inadvertently injecting the local anaesthetic into the systemic circulation, causing local anaesthetic toxicity
- allergic reaction to the local anaesthetic agent
- development of a haematoma at the site of the local anaesthetic injection (very rare)
- development of an infection (very rare).

If a block fails, always have a plan B available (e.g. conducting GA).

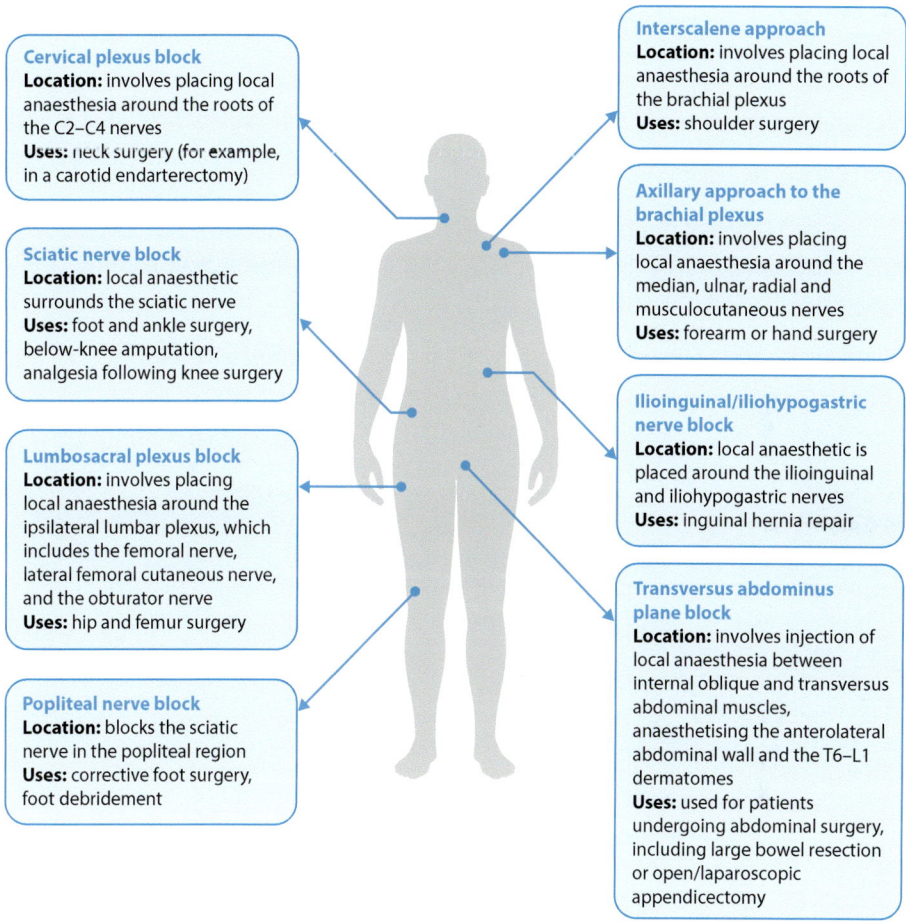

Cervical plexus block
Location: involves placing local anaesthesia around the roots of the C2–C4 nerves
Uses: neck surgery (for example, in a carotid endarterectomy)

Sciatic nerve block
Location: local anaesthetic surrounds the sciatic nerve
Uses: foot and ankle surgery, below-knee amputation, analgesia following knee surgery

Lumbosacral plexus block
Location: involves placing local anaesthesia around the ipsilateral lumbar plexus, which includes the femoral nerve, lateral femoral cutaneous nerve, and the obturator nerve
Uses: hip and femur surgery

Popliteal nerve block
Location: blocks the sciatic nerve in the popliteal region
Uses: corrective foot surgery, foot debridement

Interscalene approach
Location: involves placing local anaesthesia around the roots of the brachial plexus
Uses: shoulder surgery

Axillary approach to the brachial plexus
Location: involves placing local anaesthesia around the median, ulnar, radial and musculocutaneous nerves
Uses: forearm or hand surgery

Ilioinguinal/iliohypogastric nerve block
Location: local anaesthetic is placed around the ilioinguinal and iliohypogastric nerves
Uses: inguinal hernia repair

Transversus abdominus plane block
Location: involves injection of local anaesthesia between internal oblique and transversus abdominal muscles, anaesthetising the anterolateral abdominal wall and the T6–L1 dermatomes
Uses: used for patients undergoing abdominal surgery, including large bowel resection or open/laparoscopic appendicectomy

Figure 7.2: Location of nerve blocks that can be used in regional anaesthesia.

7.2 Neuraxial anaesthesia

Neuraxial anaesthesia is a commonly utilised, effective and safe form of regional anaesthesia. The technique involves placement of local anaesthetic (usually bupivacaine) around the spinal cord and/or the spinal nerve roots.

The two types of neuraxial anaesthesia are epidural anaesthesia (*Section 7.3*) and spinal anaesthesia (*Section 7.4*). They differ in anatomical region and equipment required.

Contraindications to neuraxial anaesthesia (both epidural and spinal anaesthesia)

Absolute:

- patient refusal
- patient allergy
- anticoagulation.

Relative:

- raised ICP
- anticoagulation
- sepsis.

7.3 Epidural anaesthesia

Epidural anaesthesia involves the injection of local anaesthetic into the epidural space. The epidural space is located between the ligamentum flavum and the dura mater. The dura mater is important anatomically in this instance, because an epidural injection does not pierce the dura, whereas spinal anaesthesia injection does (see *Figure 7.3*).

After the needle enters the epidural space, a catheter is placed into that plane in order to provide the patient with a continuous supply of local anaesthetic agent and therefore continuous analgesia or anaesthesia.

Epidural anaesthesia can also be performed with local anaesthetic combined with adjuncts (e.g. opioids such as fentanyl), and the additional opiate enhances the anaesthetic and analgesic effect.

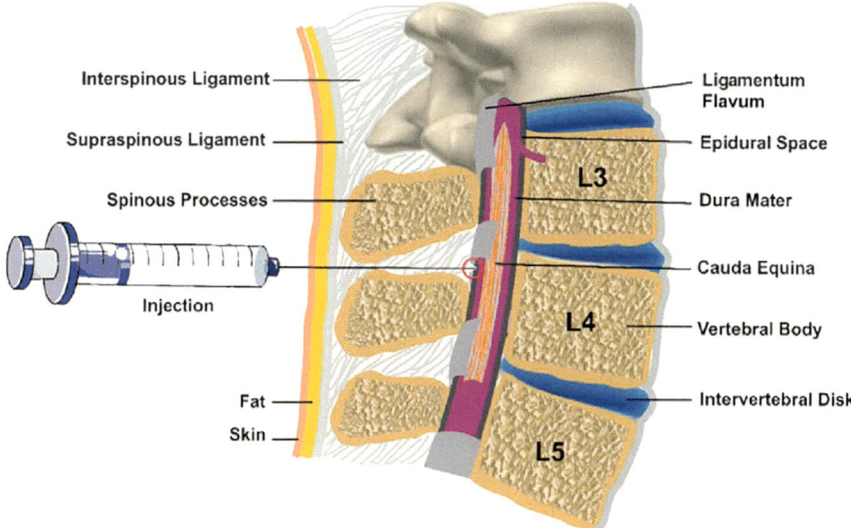

Figure 7.3: The epidural space, showing where local anaesthesia is injected in order to achieve epidural anaesthesia.

7.3.1 Clinical uses of epidural anaesthesia

Procedures

Use lumbar epidural anaesthesia to provide analgesia/anaesthesia during procedures that involve:

- childbirth
- lower limbs

- pelvis
- perineum
- abdomen.

The epidural space runs from the foramen magnum to the distal end of the spinal column and therefore is theoretically accessible at any point along this course (see *Figure 7.3*). Generally, lumbar epidurals sited between the L3 and L5 vertebrae are the most commonly used and are considered the safest because they are below the level of the spinal cord. Thoracic epidurals are used for major abdominal and chest/lung surgery. Cervical epidurals are rare but may be seen in chronic pain settings.

When used (often in the context of childbirth but also for lower limb operations), it is possible to use an epidural as the sole anaesthetic technique.

Analgesia

Epidurals are highly effective for perioperative analgesia. Intraoperatively they reduce the sympathetic response to pain, and postoperatively they can reduce PONV, and may allow for earlier discharge.

An epidural can either be continuous, with an ongoing rate of local anaesthetic delivery determined by the anaesthetist, or patient-controlled through a simple demand controller. This is where a set volume is delivered to the patient whenever the patient presses the demand button. When the maximum safe volume is delivered, this locks out and no further doses can be given to the patient. This is known as patient-controlled epidural anaesthesia (PCEA).

7.3.2 Complications of epidural anaesthesia

There are several complications that can arise from the administration of epidural anaesthesia. It must always be administered in clinical areas where resuscitation facilities are present.

Hypotension

- This is the most common adverse effect from epidural anaesthesia. The administration of local anaesthesia to the epidural space leads to the blockade of the sympathetic chain, causing peripheral vasodilatation and hypotension. In the awake state, any hypotension experienced post-insertion can result in vasovagal signs/symptoms such as dizziness, fainting, nausea and vomiting.
- Stopping the epidural infusion, lying the patient down, elevating the legs and administering an IV fluid bolus are the first steps in management, alongside administering oxygen.

- If the patient does not respond to these measures, vasopressors will need to be administered.

Total spinal anaesthesia

- Following epidural insertion, the anaesthetist performs a series of tests that help to identify that the catheter has been correctly placed within the epidural space. These tests are not 100% sensitive, and the catheter can migrate or be misplaced.
- If the epidural catheter is inserted intrathecally, i.e. the catheter lies directly around the spinal cord within the CSF, then the local anaesthetic dose delivered by the epidural route will circulate around the spinal cord to block all spinal nerve roots from C1 to S5. If the volume is sufficient, this may be enough to enter the CSF surrounding the brain, resulting in unconsciousness. This is known as a 'total spinal' and may occur in both epidural and spinal anaesthesia techniques.
- The reasons for it happening relate to patient height, positioning, level of injection and importantly the volume of local anaesthetic injected.

Initial presentation of total spinal anaesthesia includes:

- respiratory difficulty, as the diaphragm and intercostal muscles become paralysed
- arm and hand weakness
- bradycardia and arrhythmias (sympathetic cardiac accelerator fibre blockade T1–T4)
- unconsciousness as the local anaesthetic reaches the brain.

Management

This is an emergency situation and requires an immediate response. Provide the patient with the following:

1. High flow oxygen and respiratory support
2. An IV fluid bolus. Provide vasopressors for BP support.
3. If the patient has reduced Glasgow Coma Scale (GCS) score, they will require intubation and ICU admission.

The local anaesthetic will wear off over the course of a few hours and following a period of invasive ventilation on ICU, the patient should make a full recovery[42].

Dural puncture[43]

The technique of inserting an epidural means that a needle is placed close to the dura mater, and there is a risk of puncture of the dura by this needle (quoted as 1:100–500 risk). This is known as an inadvertent dural puncture.

Patients with a dural puncture can be asymptomatic, or may develop significant headache, known as a post-dural puncture headache (PDPH; see *Key notes* box below), possibly with other neurological symptoms (low CSF pressure headaches). Risk factors for a dural puncture occurring include:

- the experience of the anaesthetist
- number of attempts at epidural placement
- size of needle used (larger needles carry a bigger risk)
- young age
- pregnancy.

KEY NOTES

Post-dural puncture headache

Not all dural punctures are apparent at the time of epidural insertion, and it may be 48–72 hours after the procedure that symptoms develop.

The headache is classically postural, being worse on standing/sitting and relieved by lying down, and fronto-occipital in nature, i.e. the pain goes from the front to the back of the head.

Following presentation, it is important to first exclude other serious pathology such as venous sinus thrombosis and even meningitis, and not assume that the headache is directly caused by a dural puncture. A thorough history and examination, including a neurological examination, is paramount. Baseline observations and blood tests to look for signs of an infection, including FBC, C-reactive protein (CRP), clotting profile and blood cultures, should be considered. There are two theories that are thought to explain why dural puncture results in a headache.

1. The leakage of CSF results in reduced CSF pressure, causing traction between the brain and the skull. This causes pain and the resulting headache for the patient.
2. Due to the leakage, the drop in CSF pressure results in vasodilatation of the cerebral blood vessels, which itself results in a headache.

Management

If the diagnosis of PDPH has been made, initial management is conservative.

- Optimising hydration status, encouraging the patient to mobilise as soon as they are able, whilst taking optimum analgesia, e.g. paracetamol 1 g QDS, NSAIDs and codeine together is a starting point.
- Some studies have also found caffeine to be an effective therapy. Approximately 30–60% of patients respond to this management.

If symptoms continue or worsen over a few days instead of showing daily improvement, the next step is to offer an epidural blood patch. This involves the following steps:

1. Reinserting the epidural needle at the site of the previous epidural or an adjacent intervertebral space in a sterile manner.
2. Drawing up 20–30 ml of blood from the patient in a sterile manner from a different site (e.g. the arm).
3. Injecting this blood into the epidural space, through the sited needle, with resolution of the headache being an indicator of when to stop injecting the blood. The injection would also be stopped if discomfort increases.

It is thought that the blood will clot around the dural puncture and seal the defect. Around 70% of patients get resolution of their symptoms. If symptoms persist then a second blood patch may be offered, and if this still does not help, then discussion with a neurosurgeon is warranted.

Contraindications to administering a blood patch include:

- patients with neurological symptoms which have not been investigated
- septic patients
- patients with coagulopathy (due to the risk of haematoma formation at the site of the epidural blood patch procedure).

Epidural haematoma

Insertion or removal of the epidural may result in bleeding into the epidural space, especially in thrombocytopenic and coagulopathic patients or those on antiplatelet/anticoagulant medication.

This epidural haematoma can cause direct compression and ischaemia of the spinal cord. Patients present with lower limb weakness, paralysis and sensory block which is either more profound than that expected from the epidural anaesthetic or persists after the epidural has been removed/stopped.

This situation is a neurosurgical emergency, and urgent magnetic resonance imaging (MRI) should be arranged alongside discussion with the nearest spinal surgical centre to arrange decompression, as the patient is at risk of permanent neurological injury if not treated promptly.

7.4 Spinal anaesthesia

Spinal anaesthetic techniques deposit local anaesthetic (usually bupivacaine) inside the CSF and around the spinal cord (in the subarachnoid space) (*Figure 7.4*).

Spinal anaesthetics are usually single injections, with no catheter placement. A single injection spinal anaesthetic lasts between 2 and 4 hours and provides a profound motor and sensory block, meaning that patients are completely unable to move their legs for the duration of the local anaesthetic action (whereas it is unusual to get a complete motor block with an epidural used for analgesia)[44].

Spinal anaesthesia should be below the level of the spinal cord (below L2 vertebrae) with the L3–L4 space used preferentially because it is the most identifiable level, palpable in line with the iliac crests (in order to avoid direct spinal cord injury with a spinal needle).

Spinal anaesthesia is used in:

- obstetrics for operative delivery
- elective and emergency surgery to the lower limb
- elective and emergency urology and gynaecology surgery
- elective and emergency abdominal surgery.

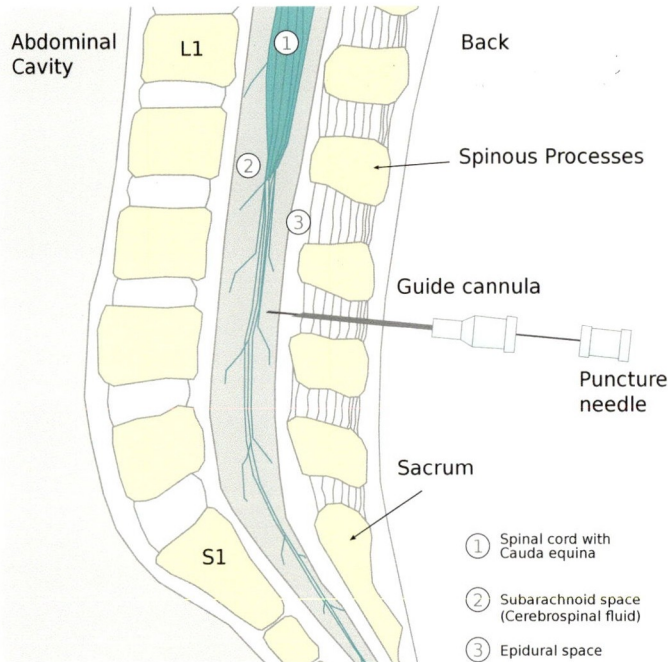

Figure 7.4: Positioning and insertion of the needle when administering local anaesthetic for spinal anaesthesia.

Contraindications to neuraxial anaesthesia:

- As discussed in *Section 7.2*.

7.4.1 Complications of spinal anaesthesia

Complications of spinal anaesthesia are shown below, from most to least common:

1. **Hypotension:** the local anaesthetic antagonises sympathetic tone, and this results in peripheral vasodilatation and hypotension. Remember that mean arterial pressure (i.e. blood pressure) is formed from cardiac output multiplied by the systemic vascular resistance (SVR). Therefore, treatment of the hypotension is aimed at increasing SVR, not cardiac output. While a fluid bolus can be given during assessment (500 ml), primary treatment involves influencing the SVR by ensuring euvolaemic status and providing vasopressors.
2. **Urinary retention:** postoperative urinary retention, and the risk factors for it developing, are described in *Section 8.2.2*.
3. **Total spinal anaesthesia:** the presentation and management of this condition is described in *Section 7.3.2*.
4. **Damage to neurological structures:** direct damage to the spinal cord or the nerve roots is rare, with an incidence of around 1:250 000. Presentation may be sensory, motor or both, involving a single spinal nerve distribution or multiple spinal nerves. These presentations are usually temporary and resolve within 12 weeks[45].

CHAPTER 8

Postoperative complications

8.1	**Postoperative nausea and vomiting**	**108**
	8.1.1 Prevention of PONV	108
8.2	**Other postoperative complications**	**110**
	8.2.1 Postoperative haemorrhage	110
	8.2.2 Postoperative urinary retention	111
8.3	**Postoperative pyrexia**	**113**
	8.3.1 Postoperative pneumonia	114
	8.3.2 Pulmonary atelectasis	115
	8.3.3 Surgical site infection	115
	8.3.4 Anastomotic leak	116
	8.3.5 Deep vein thrombosis and venous thromboembolism	117
	8.3.6 Postoperative pulmonary embolism	121

8.1 Postoperative nausea and vomiting

Up to 20% of patients receiving GA experience postoperative nausea and vomiting (PONV), defined as vomiting within 24 hours of undergoing a surgical procedure.

The risk of developing PONV is influenced by patient, anaesthetic and surgical factors[46, 47]. Patient factors that are known to increase the risk of developing PONV include:

- female gender: this is the strongest predictor of PONV
- age: younger patients are at an increased risk of developing PONV
- history of motion sickness
- non-smoking.

Anaesthetic factors that are known to increase the risk of PONV include:

- use of inhaled GA agents: risk increases in a dose-dependent manner
- use of nitrous oxide
- intraoperative and postoperative opioid use.

Surgical factors that increase PONV risk:

- gynaecology surgery
- ENT surgery
- bariatric surgery.

8.1.1 Prevention of PONV

The Apfel score may be used to stratify patients to their expected risk of suffering from PONV (see *Table 8.1*). This will allow the anaesthetist to plan perioperative anti-emetic dosage to reduce this risk as much as possible[48, 49].

Table 8.1: Patient characteristics used in the Apfel criteria

Risk factors	Points
Female	1
Non-smoker	1
History of PONV and/or motion sickness	1
Postoperative opioid administration	1

Each of these risk factors is thought to increase the incidence of PONV by 20% (i.e. a score of 3 means that the patient has a 60% risk of PONV occurring).

Anti-emetic strategies

Anti-emetic strategies are multimodal. Keeping the patient starved, adequately hydrated and normothermic preoperatively reduces the risk of PONV. If medications are required (based on the Apfel score or the patient's history):

- intraoperative doses of ondansetron 4 mg with dexamethasone 4–8 mg on induction are frequently used
- postoperative doses of ondansetron 4 mg TDS and cyclizine 50 mg TDS can be given to control PONV in the postoperative period.

In patients who have had significant PONV despite previous best efforts, avoid inhaled anaesthesia agents and offer the patient either a regional anaesthetic if appropriate or a general anaesthetic using TIVA (as propofol possesses anti-emetic properties).

8.2 Other postoperative complications

It is inevitable that some patients will experience undesired consequences and complications after surgery. As a foundation doctor you may be the first port of call to address patient and nursing concerns, and to arrange further treatment. Some issues may be simple to sort out, but other more complex problems should be escalated early so that the senior doctors may effectively manage them.

8.2.1 Postoperative haemorrhage

Any operation will cause bleeding, but haemostasis is usually accomplished by the end of surgery. If a patient is bleeding postoperatively, prompt review is required[50]. Haemorrhage is classified depending on the timing:

- Primary haemorrhage: bleeding that can be managed intraoperatively, or within the first 24 hours after surgery. Usually due to vascular injury (venous or arterial).
- Secondary haemorrhage: bleeding that occurs 7–10 days after the operation. This is often due to a wound infection.

If the bleeding is severe, it will lead to haemorrhagic shock – when blood loss is so severe that end-organ perfusion is affected. Features of postoperative haemorrhage include:

- changes in cardiovascular physiology:
  - tachycardia
  - reduced BP
  - pallor
  - weak pulse.
- secondary organ dysfunction:
  - dizziness
  - confusion
  - reduced urine output.

Management

If a patient has signs or symptoms of ongoing bleeding, severe haemorrhage or haemorrhagic shock, then a major haemorrhage call should be made to the blood bank.

As part of this major haemorrhage call, blood products will be sent to you. While awaiting this, carry out the following steps:

- Provide 500 ml boluses of crystalloid (e.g. Hartmann's solution or 0.9% saline)
- Aim for a systolic blood pressure of 90–100 mmHg – aim to be below normal systolic BP because this balances organ perfusion without increasing bleeding.

Once blood products arrive, provide the patient with packed red cells. Discuss with the on-call haematologist whether other blood products (e.g. platelets) are required.

Experienced surgical and anaesthetic assessment will determine if the patient needs to return to the operating theatre, or if they require interventional radiology for embolisation techniques.

8.2.2 Postoperative urinary retention

Postoperative urinary retention (POUR)[51] is defined as the inability to urinate after surgery despite having a full bladder. It causes significant distress to the patient, but in some patient cohorts it may go undetected.

Presenting features:

- Pain and therefore tachycardia and increased BP
- Bladder spasm
- Urinary leakage
- Large bladder palpable above the symphysis pubis.

POUR can be extremely distressing for patients, and the autonomic response to a full bladder can result in PONV, hypo-/hypertension and cardiac dysrhythmia, all of which affect postoperative recovery.

Common causes of POUR are:

- **Drugs** – some of the medications used in anaesthesia are known to affect the neurological function of the bladder. These medications include:
  - GA agents – these relax smooth muscle, thus resulting in an increase in the bladder capacity. This causes patients to have a full bladder that cannot empty effectively.
  - Neuraxial anaesthesia inhibits the sacral nerves (S2–S4) innervating the bladder, and affects the micturition reflex. Epidural anaesthesia is more commonly implicated over spinal, and so with any epidural anaesthesia we provide the patient with a urinary catheter pre-emptively. This is not required in spinal anaesthesia because its effects wear off quickly.
- **Postoperative pain** – postoperative pain activates the patient's sympathetic nervous system, which results in the contraction of the bladder sphincter, preventing micturition.

Investigating urinary retention

Conduct a bladder scan, which is an ultrasound-based assessment of the volume of fluid present within the bladder. A volume of urine in the bladder of >400 ml indicates POUR.

Management

In all cases of POUR, the bladder needs to be drained and therefore a urethral catheter must be inserted.

- If POUR is related to pain, also manage the patient's pain appropriately.
- Aside from in/out bladder drainage, if a catheter is left *in situ*, after 24–72 hours the patient can be trialled without a catheter.
- If the patient is still in retention, discuss with on-call urology, as further investigations may be required.

8.3 Postoperative pyrexia

A postoperative patient who spikes a temperature of >37.5°C should always be examined and subsequently investigated to identify the underlying cause.

There are several differentials to consider for such a temperature spike. Stratify the differentials by considering how many days after surgery the temperature spike has occurred (remember these as the **5 Ws**):

- Days 1–2: a **W**ind cause (e.g. hospital-acquired pneumonia or aspiration pneumonia, atelectasis)
- Days 3–5: a **W**ater cause (e.g. a urinary tract infection)
- Days 5–7: a **W**ound cause (e.g. a surgical site infection or deeper infective collection)
- Days 5–10: a **W**alking-related cause (e.g. the formation of a DVT, with a potential VTE)
- Any other time: **W**hat drugs and IV lines are present? Could a drug or the surgical stress response be causing the recorded pyrexia?

While these are the average number of days postoperatively that we would expect these pyrexia-causing complications to occur, this is only a guide and any of these causes could occur at any time.

In 40% of cases, the postoperative pyrexia is due to an infective cause. If an infective cause is suspected, then consider the sepsis criteria. These patients should receive sepsis management which involves the '3 in, 3 out' rules as part of the Sepsis 6 national policy (see *Table 8.2*).

Table 8.2: Sepsis 6: '3 in, 3 out' management strategy for patients with suspected sepsis

3 in	3 out
IV fluids (give 500 ml stat – but may consider 250 ml in advanced heart failure)	Peripheral blood cultures (these should be done prior to commencing antibiotics)
IV antibiotics (given in accordance with Trust policy)	Arterial lactate
Administer oxygen (aim for saturations >94%; if COPD, aim for 88–92%)	Measure urine output with a fluid chart (may require a urinary catheter to measure the fluid output)

As well as commencing sepsis management, an investigation as to the source of the infection should also be conducted. This includes the following steps:

- Requesting a chest X-ray.
- Sending the urine for culture.
- Conducting an examination of the patient, looking for evidence of pressure sores or local areas of infection, e.g. infected IV lines. If infected IV access or other foreign material (e.g. skin staples) are the likely cause of sepsis, they must be removed and re-sited as appropriate.
- Pyrexia can also be a response to inflammation, subsequent to a surgical procedure. Examples of ongoing inflammation which will need careful management include bowel anastomosis dehiscence, haematoma formation and pleural effusion.

8.3.1 Postoperative pneumonia

Postoperative pneumonia can develop in the first few days after an operation.

Pneumonia can either be a hospital-acquired pneumonia (HAP) (defined as the presence of a respiratory infection >48 hours after admission into hospital) or a community-acquired pneumonia (CAP) (defined as the presence of a respiratory infection <48 hours after admission into hospital). Aspiration pneumonitis is rare in clinical practice postoperatively.

Risk factors for developing HAP postoperatively are:

- age (risk greater with increasing age)
- smoking history
- concurrent respiratory disease
- reduced mobility postoperatively and hence reduced respiratory excursion
- immunosuppression
- diabetes
- sputum retention
- mechanical ventilation
- duration of hospital stay.

Investigations

Investigations required include:

- chest X-ray
- bloods (FBC, urea and electrolytes (U&Es), CRP) and arterial blood gas (ABG)
- sputum and blood cultures.

Management

Hypoxia should be managed with oxygen titrated to maintain saturations >94%. IV fluid resuscitation and maintenance may be required. Antibiotics are vital and the patient should complete the advised course – local guidelines will determine which antibiotic is required. Typical regimens may include the following:

If the pneumonia is not severe: doxycycline 200 mg PO stat and then 100 mg PO BD.

- If there is an aspiration pneumonia: add metronidazole 400 mg PO TDS to the doxycycline (to cover anaerobic bacteria from gut contents).

If the pneumonia is severe: co-amoxiclav 1.2 g IV TDS.

- If the patient is penicillin-allergic, provide levofloxacin 500 mg IV BD + metronidazole 400 mg PO TDS (metronidazole is only included if the patient has aspiration pneumonia).

8.3.2 Pulmonary atelectasis

Another respiratory cause of postoperative pyrexia is pulmonary atelectasis (see *Section 5.3*).

8.3.3 Surgical site infection

A surgical site infection (SSI)[52] is defined as one that occurs within 30 days of surgery around the surgical incision. The infection is typically caused by endogenous skin organisms (e.g. *Staphylococcus aureus*). Approximately 5% of patients develop an SSI after an operative procedure.

Avoiding the risk of SSIs

There are several preventative measures we implement to avoid the risk of SSIs. We can stratify these as preoperative, intraoperative or postoperative (*Table 8.3*).

Table 8.3: Preoperative, intraoperative and postoperative measures to avoid the risk of SSIs (see www.nice.org.uk/guidance/ng125/chapter/Recommendations#intraoperative-phase)

Preoperative	Patients to shower prior to operative procedure (sometimes with chlorhexidine) All staff should wear specific non-sterile theatre wear in all areas where operations are undertaken Prophylactic antibiotics to be administered to patient
Intraoperative	Surgeons to appropriately wash their hands Apply antiseptic to skin (shave area where appropriate) Maintain normothermia and adequate O_2 saturation
Postoperative	Use sterile saline for wound cleansing up to 48 hours after surgery Advise patients that they may shower safely 48 hours after surgery

Presentation

The typical features of an SSI include the following (see *Figure 8.1*):

- Pain localised to the region of the wound
- Erythema around the wound site
- Discharge at the wound site
- Breakdown of the skin.

Management

Take swabs at the infected wound site to determine the underlying pathogen of the SSI and allow the prescription of appropriate antibiotics.

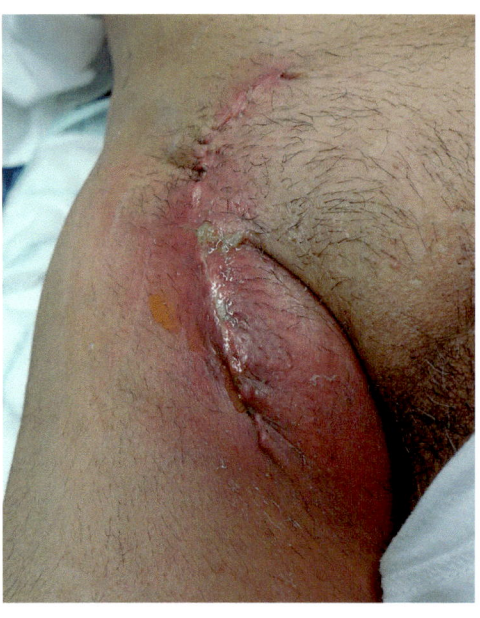

Figure 8.1: Erythema, discharge and breakdown of skin surrounding the incision site – these are the typical features of an SSI. This is an image of an SSI after a right femoral thromboendarterectomy[53].

- While awaiting these swab results, commence empirical antibiotics (flucloxacillin 500 mg PO QDS).
- Any sutures/clips at the wound site must be removed and pus must be drained from the site. The infected wound should be cleaned regularly with sterile water, and dressed appropriately (the dressing should not be so tight that it impairs blood supply to the wound).

8.3.4 Anastomotic leak

An anastomotic leak[54] occurs when there is leakage of fluid content from an intestinal anastomosis. The leaked fluid can collect within the abdominal or thoracic cavity. This complication occurs in up to 20% of bowel resection surgeries and is associated with a mortality rate of up to 40%.

The most significant risk factor for an anastomotic leak is the level of the anastomosis, with a higher rate of leaks occurring for those attempted within 7 cm of the anal verge or at the oesophagus.

Typically, anastomotic leaks present around 5–7 days post-surgery with the following symptoms and signs:

- Fever
- Oliguria
- Diarrhoea
- Localised peritonitis.

As a general rule, any patient with signs of sepsis or who is deteriorating clinically after intestinal or oesophageal surgery should always be considered to potentially have an anastomotic leak.

Investigations

An anastomotic leak is identified with a contrast CT scan (gold standard test). This will identify the presence and potential location of the leak. Other investigations to conduct include:

- repeat bloods: FBC, CRP and blood cultures (to exclude other causes of sepsis)
- a venous blood gas to determine the blood lactate (to rule out ischaemic bowel).

Management

A patient with a suspected anastomotic leak requires an urgent senior review.

- All patients must be made nil by mouth (NBM) and commenced on broad-spectrum antibiotics (as per the local protocol) to reduce the risk of infection from the leaked bowel contents.
- Commence IV fluids and monitor urine output (insert a catheter).

Further management depends on the extent of the leak and the fitness of the patient.

- If the leak, as identified by the contrast CT scan, is small then conservative management with IV antibiotics is appropriate.
- However, if the leak is large but localised, then percutaneous drainage is required to remove the fluid.
- If percutaneous drainage fails or the patient is septic or has multiple collections throughout the abdomen, then an exploratory laparotomy is required to wash out the collections and to place a drain into the abdomen to allow continued drainage and prevent the re-accumulation of intestinal contents.

8.3.5 Deep vein thrombosis and venous thromboembolism

The way in which surgery increases the risk of a DVT forming is discussed in *Section 2.6*. If a DVT/VTE occurs, it typically presents 5–10 days postoperatively.

Deep vein thrombosis

A DVT is when a thrombus (blood clot) forms in the deep veins of the upper or lower limbs.

Risk factors for DVT formation include the following (remember these by the mnemonic **THROMBOSIS**):

- **T**ravel (particularly long journeys that involve immobility)
- **H**ypercoagulable blood / **H**ormone replacement therapy containing oestrogens
- **R**ecreational drug use
- **O**lder age (>60 years)
- **M**alignancy
- **B**irth control pill (containing oestrogens)
- **O**besity / **O**bstetric patients
- **S**urgery/**S**moking
- **I**mmobilisation
- **S**ickness (e.g. chronic heart, liver or kidney disease).

A DVT is classified as being 'provoked' if there is a distinct underlying cause (e.g. underlying malignancy). If no cause can be identified for the DVT, then it is classified as being 'unprovoked'.

Presentation

If a DVT develops after surgery, it will typically present around days 5–10. Presenting symptoms depend on the size and the location of the blood clot. If the clot is small, the patient may be asymptomatic. This is common and an estimated 50% of patients with a DVT have no symptoms. Larger clots present with:

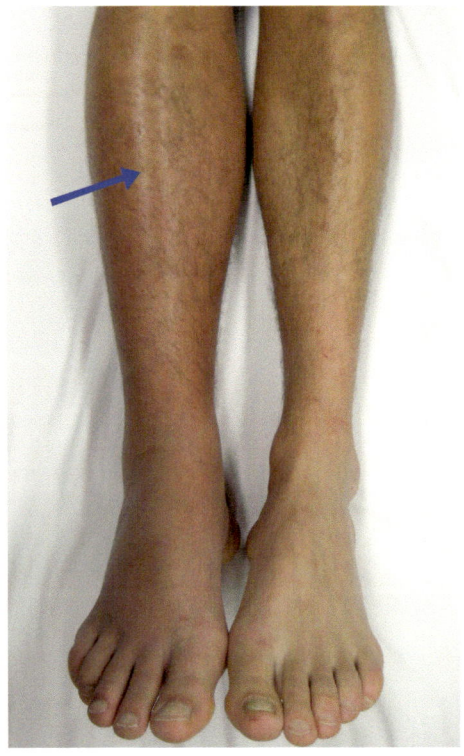

- pain and swelling at the location of the DVT (*Figure 8.2*)
- fever
- pain in the calf when the toes and foot are stretched upwards (called 'Homans sign').

Figure 8.2: A DVT of the right calf.

Investigations

If the patient has symptoms of a DVT, NICE recommends using the two-level Wells score (see *Table 8.4*) to determine subsequent appropriate investigations[55].

Table 8.4: The two-level Wells score for determining the risk of DVT[56]

Clinical feature	Points
Active cancer (treatment ongoing, within 6 months, or palliative)	1
Paralysis, paresis, or recent plaster immobilisation of the lower extremities	1
Recently bedridden >3 days or major surgery within 12 weeks requiring general or regional anaesthesia	1
Localised tenderness along the distribution of the deep venous system	1
Entire leg swollen	1
Calf swelling 3 cm larger than asymptomatic side	1
Pitting oedema confined to the symptomatic leg	1
Collateral superficial veins (non-varicose)	1
Previously documented DVT	1
Alternative diagnosis at least as likely as DVT	−2

Based on this scoring system, consider:

- a DVT to be likely if the patient scores ≥2 points
- a DVT to be unlikely if the patient scores ≤1 point.

The definitive test to identify a DVT is with an ultrasound scan of the calf and suspected veins. NICE recommends offering patients with a 'likely' two-level Wells score either of the following:

- A leg vein Doppler USS. This should be conducted within 4 hours of being requested and, if the result is negative, a D-dimer test should be conducted to be certain that a DVT is not present.
- If a leg vein ultrasound cannot be conducted within 4 hours, then request a D-dimer test and provide therapeutic anticoagulation, e.g. enoxaparin 1 mg/kg actual body weight BD until the ultrasound has been performed.

If the patient has an 'unlikely' two-level Wells score, conduct a D-dimer test only; if the result is positive, treat the patient as being 'likely' to have a DVT and arrange a subsequent leg USS.

> ### KEY NOTES
>
> #### What is a D-dimer test?
>
> D-dimer is a protein that is produced when a blood clot is formed. With a large clot (as seen in a DVT), abnormally raised levels of D-dimer can be identified within the blood. A raised D-dimer is *sensitive*, but not *specific*, for a DVT: if a DVT is present, it will always cause a raised D-dimer.
>
> However, there can also be other causes of a raised D-dimer, including disseminated intravascular coagulation, being postoperative, an infection, the presence of liver disease, kidney disease, malignancy and pregnancy. This means that the D-dimer test has a low *specificity* for detecting a DVT. For this reason, do not diagnose a DVT by a raised D-dimer alone – use an ultrasound to confirm its presence.

Management

If there are no contraindications (e.g. pregnancy or cancer), a confirmed postoperative DVT is treated with an oral anticoagulant such as warfarin or apixaban. The oral anticoagulant is provided for 3 months. If providing warfarin, then aim for an INR target of 2–3.

> ### KEY NOTES
>
> #### Further investigations
>
> A postoperative DVT is considered a provoked DVT, because a cause for the condition is present. However, if no cause for the DVT can be easily identified from the patient's history, then further investigations are required.
>
> NICE recommends (NG158, 2020) the following investigations for a patient with an unprovoked DVT to exclude cancer:
>
> - a physical examination
> - a chest X-ray
> - blood tests (including FBC, serum calcium and liver function tests)
> - urinalysis
> - an abdominal–pelvic computed tomography (CT) scan (and a mammogram for women) if the patient is >40 years of age and the tests listed above have not demonstrated signs of a cancer.
>
> Furthermore, once anticoagulation has been stopped, if the DVT was unprovoked then test for antiphospholipid antibodies and hereditary thrombophilia (the latter only if the patient has a first-degree relative who has had a DVT).

8.3.6 Postoperative pulmonary embolism

Patients who develop a DVT perioperatively are at risk of developing a pulmonary embolus (PE), where a clot blocks or restricts blood flow through the pulmonary arteries. A DVT requires treatment because progression to a PE has serious consequences in terms of increased morbidity and mortality.

Massive PE is a condition that may present with significant cardiorespiratory compromise and even cardiac arrest, which requires urgent assessment and treatment by a senior clinician.

Other risk factors for a PE can include:

- hypercoagulability in the blood secondary to cancer
- a fat embolism (which can occur after a long bone fracture)
- a thrombus in the cardiac ventricles – this can develop after a myocardial infarction (rare cause)
- pregnancy
- atrial fibrillation.

Presentation

A PE is most likely to present at days 5–10 postoperatively, with typical presenting features including:

- chest pain
- dyspnoea
- tachypnoea
- pyrexia
- tachycardia
- hypotension
- hypoxia which may be refractory to oxygen therapy
- cyanosis.

The risk factors for developing a PE are the same as those for a DVT and can be remembered by the mnemonic **THROMBOSIS** (see *Section 8.3.5*). Classify a PE as being 'provoked' if any clear underlying cause is present. If there is no clear underlying cause then it is classified as being 'unprovoked'.

Investigations

Features on an ECG which are often present in patients with PE include:

- sinus tachycardia (most common)
- right bundle branch block
- right ventricular strain (causing inverted T waves in leads V_1 to V_4)
- an $S_1Q_3T_3$ pattern to the ECG; in this pattern, there is a large S wave in lead 1, a large Q wave and an inverted T wave in lead 3.

Features on a chest X-ray that indicate a PE include (*Figure 8.3*):

- the presence of a prominent pulmonary artery (Fleischner sign)
- a 'Hampton hump', which is a wedge-shaped area of pleural consolidation (whitening) in the lung fields
- the presence of Westermark sign: reduced lung markings in the area of the lungs supplied by the vessels that have been blocked by the pulmonary embolus.

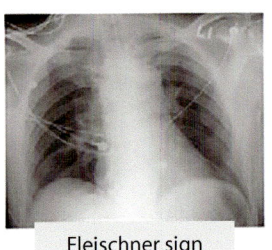
Fleischner sign

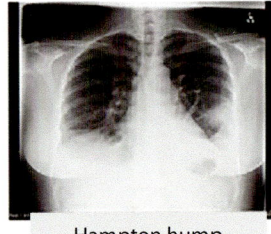
Hampton hump

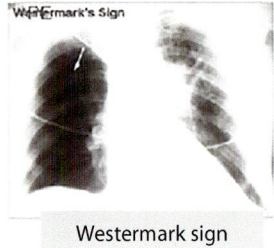
Westermark sign

Figure 8.3: Characteristic features seen in a chest X-ray with a PE[57].

Note that a chest X-ray is most likely to have a normal appearance and is not sensitive enough on its own to confirm the diagnosis of PE.

If a PE is suspected, then NICE recommends conducting a PE Wells score in order to determine whether further investigations are indicated[58]. This is similar to the two-level Wells score that is used in DVT management (see *Table 8.5*).

Table 8.5: The pulmonary embolism Wells score

Variable	Points
Clinical signs or symptoms of DVT	3.0
Alternative diagnosis less likely than PE	3.0
Heart rate >100 beats/minute	1.5
Immobilisation or surgery in previous 4 weeks	1.5
Previous VTE	1.5
Haemoptysis	1.0
Active cancer	1.0

Based on this scoring system, consider:

- a PE to be likely if the patient scores ≥5 points
- a PE to be unlikely if the patient scores ≤4 points.

If the patient's Wells score is in the 'unlikely' range, then a D-dimer test is recommended to exclude a PE. However, if the PE Wells score indicates that a PE is 'likely', then the best test is a CTPA (CT pulmonary angiogram). If this is contraindicated (e.g. the patient has poor renal function or is pregnant), then a ventilation/perfusion scan (V/Q scan) can be conducted instead.

Management

If the patient has a confirmed PE but is haemodynamically stable, then they are treated with oral anticoagulation, with enoxaparin bridging, for 3 months.

If the patient is haemodynamically unstable and a PE is suspected as the most likely cause, thrombolysis may be required, e.g. alteplase 100 mg IV administered over 2 hours. A senior clinician should make this decision, because there is mortality and morbidity associated with thrombolysis that needs to be taken into consideration.

Absolute contraindications to administering thrombolysis include the following:

- The patient having any previous haemorrhagic stroke, or an ischaemic stroke in the last 6 months
- A CNS tumour or a brain injury
- Any trauma in the last 3 weeks
- Any GI bleed in the last month
- A known bleeding risk.

If thrombolysis fails, then thrombectomy (mechanical removal of the thrombus under radiological guidance) is an alternative.

CHAPTER 9

MCQs and OSCE scenarios

9.1	MCQs	126
9.2	OSCE scenarios	129
9.3	Case-based discussions	131
	9.3.1 Left-sided primary total hip replacement	131
	9.3.2 Left inguinal hernia repair	132
	9.3.3 Total hysterectomy: open procedure	132
9.4	Answers to MCQs	134
9.5	Answers to OSCE scenarios	136

9.1 MCQs

For answers see *Section 9.4*.

1. **Which one of the following is the mechanism of action of local anaesthetics?**
   a. Binding to voltage-gated sodium channels
   b. Binding to voltage-gated calcium channels
   c. Binding to ligand-gated channels
   d. Binding to mu opioid G-protein coupled receptors

2. **A 30-year-old woman has a laceration to her finger. A digital block was done for the region; 3 ml of 1% lidocaine was used. How long will it most likely take for her to regain sensation to her finger?**
   a. 20 minutes
   b. 45 minutes
   c. 90 minutes
   d. 120 minutes

3. **A patient weighs 80 kg and requires local anaesthetic 1% lidocaine. What is the maximum dose of lidocaine that can be used?**
   a. 16 ml
   b. 20 ml
   c. 22 ml
   d. 24 ml

4. **A 70-year-old man has dislocated his right elbow, which is to be reduced under sedation. His past medical history includes stable angina and COPD. He currently smokes and has a 30 pack-year smoking history. He lives an active lifestyle and does the shopping himself. What would his ASA grade be?**
   a. 1
   b. 2
   c. 3
   d. 4
   e. 5

9.1

5. **A 30-year-old woman is receiving a local lidocaine 1% block on her finger in preparation for a tendon repair. She starts to feel some numbness in her tongue and around her mouth. Which of the following would be the most appropriate management option?**
   a. Monitor and carry on slowly
   b. Reassure her, as she could be having a panic attack
   c. Stop the procedure and give her a paper bag to rebreathe in
   d. Stop the procedure and give oxygen

6. **Lidocaine can cause all of the following except:**
   a. Sedation
   b. Convulsions
   c. Slowed A-V conduction
   d. Prolongation of the cardiac action potential
   e. Shortening of the refractory phase

7. **Below which vertebrae would the needle be safest to enter when administering spinal anaesthesia?**
   a. T11
   b. T12
   c. L1
   d. L2

8. **Which one key structure is pierced when administering local anaesthetic into the epidural space?**
   a. Dura
   b. Arachnoid mater
   c. Ligamentum flavum
   d. Pia mater

9. **Which of the following is an inhibitor of the NMDA glutamate receptor?**
   a. Thiopental
   b. Sevoflurane
   c. Halothane
   d. Ketamine

10. **Halothane can be used for both induction and maintenance of GA. Its limited use is due to which one of the following reasons?**
    a. Severe hepatotoxicity issues
    b. Long time to recover once used
    c. Bronchial and salivary secretions
    d. Slower onset of actions than other anaesthetics

11. **Which of the following is the treatment for malignant hyperthermia?**
    a. Adrenaline
    b. Lidocaine
    c. Dantrolene
    d. Bromocriptine

12. **You are asked to see a patient 1 week after their operation due to a change in their observations. They had an elective laparotomy for their Crohn's disease and now have a stoma in place. Their observations are as follows: BP 125/89, HR 105, RR 25, sats 96% on room air, temperature 37.8°C. They don't complain of any pain and their wound site looks clean. What would be the most useful investigation?**
    a. Chest X-ray
    b. Doppler USS
    c. Bloods including D-dimer
    d. Blood cultures

9.2 OSCE scenarios

We have provided two different OSCE scenarios for you to practise with. You will need a partner to properly conduct this section – one person asking the questions and the other providing the answers.

For answers see *Section 9.5*.

OSCE Station 1

Airway management

> **1. Name the airway adjuncts shown in the figure below.**
>
>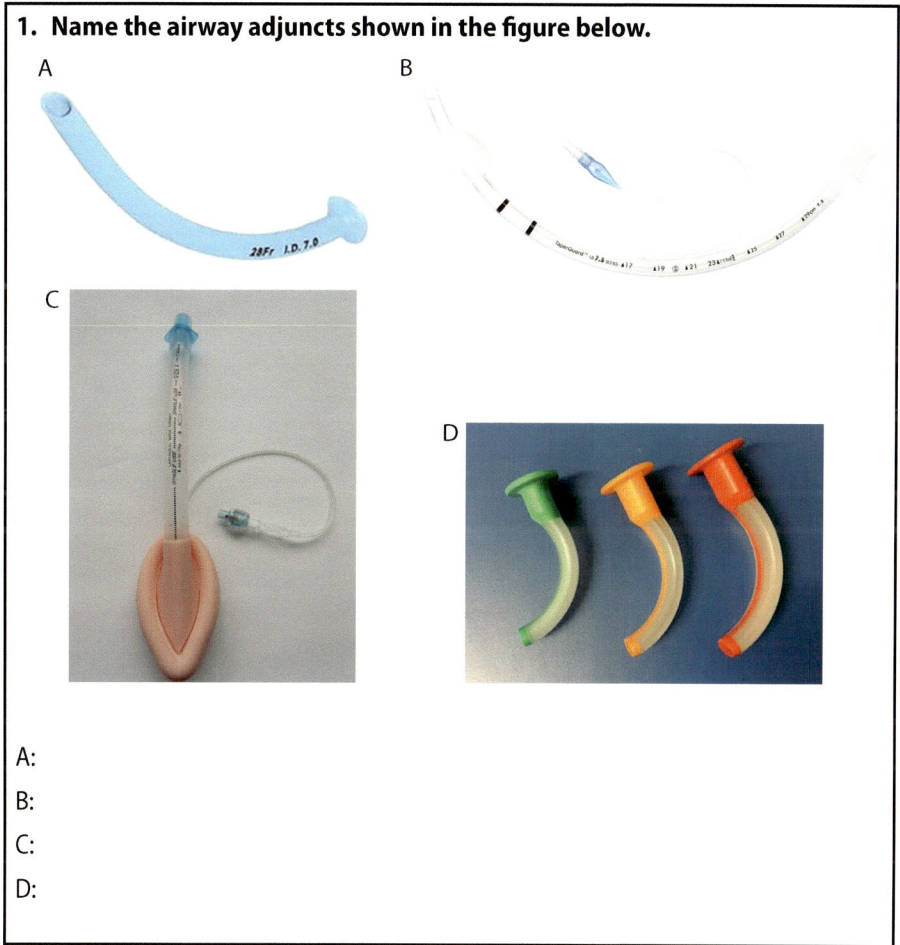
>
> A:
>
> B:
>
> C:
>
> D:

Scenario: A patient is brought to A&E by ambulance following a cycling accident. His GCS is E2 V3 M3. He arrives with an oxygen mask already on. You notice there is now reduced fogging of the facemask and it sounds as if the patient might be snoring.

2. How would you initially manage this patient?

If candidate does not mention the most appropriate airway device to use and its sizing after they discuss airway manoeuvres, please ask *Questions 3* and *4*:

3. Which airway device would be most appropriate?

4. How would you size this?

5. Can you show me how to insert this in the model please?

You have now successfully inserted the adjunct into the patient's airway. Their oxygen saturations stabilise, and chest expansion is currently equal. Their GCS score is now 9. For now, your A–E assessment is complete.

6. What would be your next step?

OSCE Station 2: Viva/discussion

Differences between LA and GA

1. Please tell me about the different types of anaesthetic techniques.

2. Name some of the different types of muscle relaxants that are available in anaesthetic practice.

Suxamethonium is a type of muscle relaxant, depolarising in nature. This is used in a patient undergoing a laparotomy and requiring GA. During the anaesthetic process, the patient's muscles appear rigid and it becomes difficult to open their jaw. You also notice, despite increased mechanical ventilation, that the patient's end-tidal carbon dioxide concentration increases.

3. What do you think is happening and how would you treat this?

9.3 Case-based discussions

To appreciate how this all comes together, we have written some cases below of common operative scenarios and what methods of anaesthesia may be used. This helps you understand how all these steps in assessing the patient come together to influence our anaesthetic choices. Not all steps to be considered are written here (e.g. blood loss group and save), but just the key points.

9.3.1 Left-sided primary total hip replacement

Preoperative assessment and planning

1. Anaesthetic history
   - 74y F
   - PMHx: hypertension, osteoarthritis
   - DHx: amlodipine 5 mg OD, paracetamol 1 g QDS, naproxen 250 mg TDS
2. Airway planning and Bloods
   - No distinct airway concerns
   - ASA grade: 2, major operation
   - FBC, U&E and ECG evaluated – all within normal limits
3. Medication management
   - NSAIDs stopped on day of surgery whilst fasting
   - Operation date organised at least 4 weeks after antibiotics stopped for a chest infection, in order to mitigate increased upper airway reactivity after lower respiratory tract infection (LRTI)
4. VTE prophylaxis
   - Intraoperatively: thromboelastic deterrent stocking and sequential compression device right leg (mechanical prophylaxis)
   - Postoperatively: LMWH for 4 weeks (chemical prophylaxis).

Choice of anaesthesia

- Mainstay anaesthesia: spinal injection with local anaesthetic and opiate
  - during spinal anaesthesia, the patient can be awake, sedated or have a general anaesthetic
- Postoperative analgesia: paracetamol, NSAID, long-acting opiate 48 h, PRN short-acting opiate; spinal opiate will contribute to analgesia for 8–16 h.

9.3.2 Left inguinal hernia repair

Preoperative assessment and planning

1. Anaesthetic history
   - 74y M
   - PMHx: atrial fibrillation
   - DHx: bisoprolol 5 mg OD, rivaroxaban 20 mg OD
2. Airway planning and Bloods
   - No distinct airway concerns
   - ASA grade: 2, intermediate operation
   - U&E and ECG evaluated – all within normal limits; coagulation also checked in this patient as currently anticoagulated
3. Medication management
   - Stop rivaroxaban for 48 h
4. VTE prophylaxis
   - Intraoperatively: thromboelastic deterrent stockings (mechanical prophylaxis)
   - Continued postoperatively (constantly under review until fully mobile)

Choice of anaesthesia

- Mainstay: local anaesthesia field block including an ilio-inguinal nerve block
- This procedure can be completed awake like this, if the patient is willing; often older patients are more tolerant as long as positioning in the supine / head up position is possible
- Alternatively, sedation with midazolam and propofol can be provided, and the patient will require extraneous oxygen
- Postoperative analgesia: paracetamol, NSAID, up to 1 week.

9.3.3 Total hysterectomy: open procedure

Preoperative assessment and planning

1. Anaesthetic history
   - 24y F
   - PMHx: mild asthma
   - DHx: salbutamol inhaler PRN
2. Airway planning and Bloods
   - No distinct airway concerns
   - ASA grade: 2, major operation
   - FBC, U&E and ECG evaluated – all within normal limits
3. Medication management
   - Nil

4. VTE prophylaxis
- Intraoperatively: thromboelastic deterrent stockings (mechanical prophylaxis)
- Continued until fully mobile.

Choice of anaesthesia

- Mainstay: spinal injection with local anaesthetic and opiate (larger volume than hip replacement therefore a higher truncal dermatomal block)
  - combined with a GA and muscle relaxation
  - PR diclofenac if tolerated
- Postoperative analgesia: paracetamol, NSAID, PRN oral opiate.

9.4 Answers to MCQs

1. **A.** Local anaesthetics work by blocking the entry of sodium ions into their channels in the neural membrane, thereby preventing depolarisation, i.e. no action potential can be propagated.

2. **B.** Usually, plain lidocaine (when adrenaline is not coupled with it) takes a couple of minutes to act, with effects lasting about 30–60 minutes. Effects are prolonged if adrenaline is used with lidocaine. Remember, however, that mixing adrenaline with lidocaine is contraindicated when administering LA to a digit, to the penis, to the nose or to the ears (due to the risk of causing local ischaemia from vasoconstriction in an extremity).

3. **D.** Remember that the dose of lidocaine is calculated per kg of body weight. The maximum dose is 3 mg/kg without adrenaline. Therefore, 3 mg × 80 kg = 240 mg. This is 24 ml as 1 mg = 0.1 ml (see *Chapter 6* on local anaesthesia).

4. **B.** ASA grade 2 means the patient has mild–moderate disease, but their normal daily activity is not limited. A useful and time-saving way to handle this question is to eliminate the last two options (d and e) and first option (a). Then remember that 3 is always the 'turning point' in activity status – i.e. ASA 3 is when a patient's severe disease limits activity. Note that pregnancy is also a criterion for ASA 2.

    ASA grades are important to ascertain the fitness of patients and are used with other factors to help describe a patient's perioperative risk.

5. **D.** Often the first symptoms or signs of LA toxicity can be neurological, such as perioral tingling, numbness or paraesthesia, slurred speech, light-headedness, tinnitus and/or confusion.

    You should stop the procedure, carry out an A–E assessment and involve your senior. Within your assessment it would be vital to maintain the airway and give the patient 100% oxygen.

    You should also monitor the patient by attaching an observation machine, and take an ECG.

6. **D.** Slowed AV conduction can lead to heart block but not due to prolongation of the cardiac action potential.

7. **D.** In most people L2 is when the spinal cord ends, and therefore usually below L2 is the safest position, as you are unlikely to hit the spinal cord.

8. **C.** Epidural anaesthesia is achieved by placing a needle (which you then remove) and leaving a catheter between the ligamentum flavum and dura mater, i.e. outside the dura mater. The ligamentum flavum is the anatomical landmark as a loss of resistance indicates that you are in the epidural space.

9.   **D.** Ketamine antagonises the NMDA receptor.

10. **A.** This is also known as halothane hepatitis.

11. **C.** Dantrolene 2 mg/kg. Dantrolene inhibits the efflux of calcium from the sarcoplasmic reticulum, thus reducing the concentration of calcium in the skeletal muscle cells and therefore ceasing the contraction.

   The administration of dantrolene should be repeated every 5 minutes until the cardiac and respiratory systems are stabilised. You should ensure the precipitating agent has been removed and the patient has 100% oxygen when carrying out an A–E assessment.

12. **A.** Chest X-ray – you are most concerned here about a PE, therefore you would want a chest X-ray in the first instance and then a CTPA. The patient could have a DVT present; however, the fact that this patient has a tachycardia and a higher respiratory rate means you should be most concerned about a PE. You would also calculate a Wells score.

   Note a D-dimer can be useful; however, post-surgery is likely to be raised anyway therefore a chest X-ray is more useful. A low-grade fever can often be seen with a PE.

9.5 Answers to OSCE scenarios

OSCE Station 1

Airway management

> **1. Name the airway adjuncts shown in the figure below.**
>
>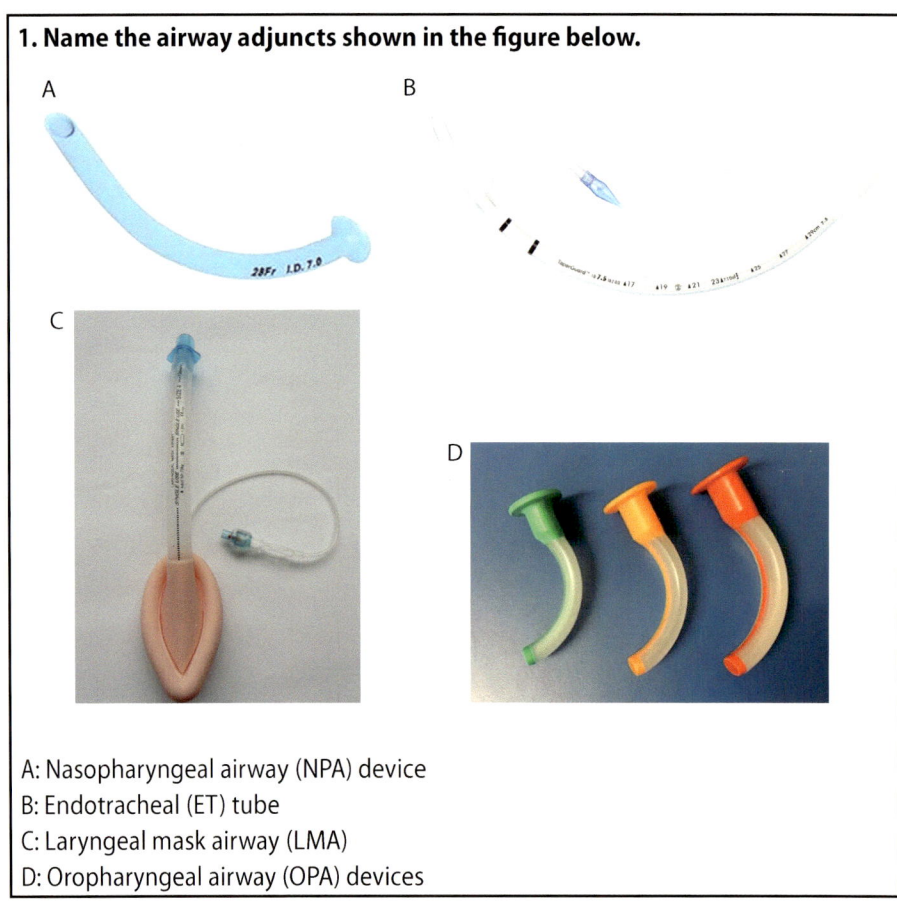
>
> A: Nasopharyngeal airway (NPA) device
> B: Endotracheal (ET) tube
> C: Laryngeal mask airway (LMA)
> D: Oropharyngeal airway (OPA) devices

Scenario: A patient is brought to A&E following a cycling accident. His GCS is E2 V3 M3. He arrives with an oxygen mask already on from the ambulance crew. You notice there is now reduced fogging of the facemask and it sounds as if the patient might be snoring.

2. How would you initially manage this patient?
Mention A–E assessment always, and call your senior.
- You are trained in basic life support (BLS), and should be trained in intermediate life support (ILS) and eventually advanced life support (ALS). Simple airway manoeuvres include head tilt–chin lift, and then progressing to a jaw thrust.
- This could be a road traffic accident (RTA), as we don't know the nature of the cycling accident from this brief history. Therefore, you should mention/ acknowledge that in trauma patients, we would do the jaw thrust not the head tilt–chin lift manoeuvre, to protect the C-spine.
- Next, you would move on to airway adjuncts. This patient has airway compromise with diminished fogging of his mask and 'snoring' sounds. His low GCS score (8) shows he is unconscious. If a patient tolerates an OPA or NPA, it tells you they're unconscious and have a vulnerable airway. These adjuncts are buying you time until an advanced practitioner arrives.

If a candidate does not mention the most appropriate airway device to use and its sizing after they discuss airway manoeuvres, please ask *Questions 3* and *4*:

3. Which airway device would be most appropriate?
Oropharyngeal airway (or Guedel).
Adjuncts such as OPA and NPA help to immediately address airway obstruction and free the airway practitioner. Both adjuncts are generally only tolerated in unconscious patients.

4. How would you size this?
Incisor to the angle of the jaw (see figure).

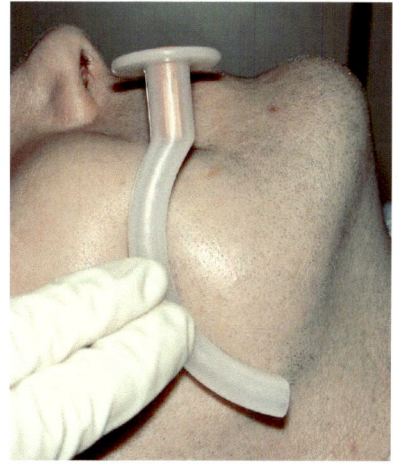

5. Can you show me how to insert this in the model please?

Insert the OPA upside down, and then once inserted halfway / behind the tongue you can turn it 180°. This way you prevent catching the tongue and obstructing the airway.

You have now successfully inserted the oropharyngeal airway (or Guedel) into the patient's airway. Their oxygen saturations stabilise, and chest expansion is currently equal. Their GCS score is now 9. For now, your A–E assessment is complete.

6. What would be your next step?

Call your senior / alert the anaesthetics registrar. If a patient is tolerating an OPA or NPA, consider the need for an advanced airway practitioner and intubation. Tolerating an OPA is an indicator of a vulnerable unprotected airway.

This is a scenario for a formal trauma call, which follows ATLS guidance. After ABC evaluation, a full physical examination including a full spinal examination for other injuries is appropriate.

Carry out investigations:
- Bedside (bloods, ABG/VBG – you would like to know the acid–base status and want a lactate)
- CT head.

Knowledge of the other injuries he may have encountered will determine what you need to order as imaging.

OSCE Station 2: Viva/discussion

Differences between LA and GA

1. Please tell me about the different types of anaesthetic techniques.

- GA is a triad of hypnosis / analgesia / muscle relaxation in order to deliver a reversible state of unconsciousness. Analgesics reduce sympathetic pain response and muscle relaxants are used in certain surgical situations (e.g. PPV).
- Regional anaesthesia interrupts nerve signals from a single nerve or group of nerves. It can be used to facilitate surgery on its own (e.g. knee replacement), in combination with GA or solely for analgesia.
- Local anaesthesia blocks nerve transmission from small nerve endings to a superficial location for a specific procedure, e.g. suturing a skin laceration.

2. Name some of the different types of muscle relaxants that are available in anaesthetic practice.

- Drugs that cause reversible skeletal muscle paralysis are known as neuromuscular blocking drugs (NMBDs). They are sometimes referred to as muscle relaxants.
- There are two types: depolarising and non-depolarising.
- Non-depolarising drugs include rocuronium, while a depolarising drug is suxamethonium.

Suxamethonium is a type of muscle relaxant, depolarising in nature. This is used in a patient undergoing a laparotomy and requiring GA. During the anaesthetic process, the patient's muscles appear rigid and it becomes difficult to open their jaw. You also notice, despite increased mechanical ventilation, that the patient's end-tidal carbon dioxide concentration increases.

3. What do you think is happening and how would you treat this?

- Malignant hyperthermia or hyperpyrexia
- Autosomal dominant condition
- Some patients have a higher risk of developing this reaction to suxamethonium
- Features include: muscle rigidity, often starting with masseter muscle rigidity, pyrexia, tachycardia, increased CO_2 production, mixed acidosis, ECG changes for hyperkalaemia.
- Lab results would show: increased creatine kinase (CK), hyperkalaemia, rhabdomyolysis, AKI, renal failure
- Treatment: dantrolene and physiology support.

References

1. Kizilbash, A. and Ngô-Minh, C.T. (2014) Review of extended-release formulations of Tramadol for the management of chronic non-cancer pain: focus on marketed formulations. *J Pain Res*, **7:** 149–61.

2. NICE (2016) *Routine preoperative tests for elective surgery* [NG45]. Available from: www.nice.org.uk/guidance/ng45.

3. NICE/BNF *Diabetes, surgery and medical illness*. Available from: https://bnf.nice.org.uk/treatment-summary/diabetes-surgery-and-medical-illness.html.

4. Whittington Health (2012, reviewed 2015) *Steroid dependent patients who are undergoing surgery or are acutely unwell.*

5. Hoogendoorn, C.J., Roy, J.F. and Gonzalez, J.S. (2017) Shared dysregulation of homeostatic brain-body pathways in depression and type 2 diabetes. *Curr Diab Rep*, **17(10):** 90.

6. Keeling, D., Tait, R.C., Watson, H. and British Committee of Standards for Haematology (2016) Peri-operative management of anticoagulation and antiplatelet therapy. *Br J Haematol*, **175(4):** 602–13.

7. NICE (2018, revised 2022) *Contraception – combined hormonal methods.* Available from: https://cks.nice.org.uk/contraception-combined-hormonal-methods#!scenario.

8. Steeds, C. and Orme, R. (2006) Premedication. *Anaesthesia & Intensive Care Medicine*, **7(11):** 393–6.

9. NICE (2019, revised 2022) *Scenario: Management of deep vein thrombosis.* Available from: https://cks.nice.org.uk/topics/deep-vein-thrombosis/management/management.

10. NICE (2018, updated 2019) *Venous thromboembolism in over 16s: reducing the risk of hospital-acquired deep vein thrombosis or pulmonary embolism* [NG89] Available from www.nice.org.uk/guidance/NG89.

11. Dennis, M., Sandercock, P., Reid, J. *et al.* (2013) Effectiveness of intermittent pneumatic compression in reduction of risk of deep vein thrombosis in patients who have had a stroke (CLOTS 3): a multicentre randomised controlled trial. *Lancet*, **382(9891):** 516–24.

12. Smith, I., Kranke, P., Murat, I. *et al.* (2011) Perioperative fasting in adults and children: guidelines from the European Society of Anaesthesiology. *Eur J Anaesthesiol*, **28(8):** 556–69.

13. Sellers, C. and Woodman, N. (2023) Inhalational induction in paediatric anaesthesia. *BJA Education*, **23(1):** 32–8.

14. Sajayan, A., Wicker, J., Ungureanu, N. *et al.* (2016) Current practice of rapid sequence induction of anaesthesia in the UK – a national survey. *Br J Anaesth*, 117 Suppl 1: i69–i74.

15. NICE (2012) *Depth of anaesthesia monitors – Bispectral Index (BIS), E-Entropy and Narcotrend-Compact M.* [DG6]

16. Tsukamoto, M., Taura, S., Yamanaka, H. *et al.* (2020) Age-related effects of

three inhalational anesthetics at one minimum alveolar concentration on electroencephalogram waveform. *Aging Clin Exp Res*, **32(9):** 1857–64.

17. Ljungqvist, O., Scott, M. and Fearon, K.C. (2017) Enhanced recovery after surgery: a review. *JAMA Surg*, **152(3):** 292–8.

18. Elbaih, A.H. and Basyouni, F.H. (2020) Teaching approach of primary survey in trauma patients. *Int J Intern Emerg Med*, **3(3):** 1035.

19. Sampson, M. (2021) A guide to airway management. *British Journal of Cardiac Nursing*, **16(3):** 1–13.

20. Goudra, B. and Singh, P.M. (2017) Airway management during upper GI endoscopic procedures: state of the art review. *Dig Dis Sci*, **62(1):** 45–53.

21. Santillanes, G. and Gausche-Hill, M. (2008) Pediatric airway management. *Emerg Med Clin N Am*, **26(4):** 961–975.

22. Keller, C., Brimacombe, J. and Benzer, A. (1999) Calculated vs measured pharyngeal mucosal pressures with the laryngeal mask airway during cuff inflation: assessment of four locations. *Br J Anaesth*, **82(3):** 399–401.

23. Smith, S.L. and Thomson, S.L. (2013) Influence of subglottic stenosis on the flow-induced vibration of a computational vocal fold model. *J Fluids Struct*, **38:** 77–91.

24. Ruetzler, K., Smereka, J., Abelairas-Gomez, C. *et al.* (2020) Comparison of the new flexible tip bougie catheter and standard bougie stylet for tracheal intubation by anesthesiologists in different difficult airway scenarios: a randomized crossover trial. *BMC Anesthesiology*, **20(1):** 90.

25. Ruetzler, K., Szarpak, L., Smereka, J. *et al.* (2020) Comparison of direct and video laryngoscopes during different airway scenarios performed by experienced paramedics: a randomized cross-over manikin study. *BioMed Research International*, **2020:** 5382739.

26. Ansari, L., Bohluli, B., Mahaseni, H. *et al.* (2014) The effect of endotracheal tube cuff pressure control on postextubation throat pain in orthognathic surgeries: a randomized double-blind controlled clinical trial. *British Journal of Oral and Maxillofacial Surgery*, **52(2):** 140–143.

27. Flin, R., Patey, R., Glavin, R. and Maran, N. (2010) Anaesthetists' non-technical skills. *Br J Anaesth*, **105(1):** 38–44.

28. Difficult Airway Society (2015) *DAS guidelines for management of unanticipated difficult intubation in adults*. Reproduced with permission of the Difficult Airway Society.

29. Harper, N.J., Cook, T.M., Garcez, T. *et al.* (2018) Anaesthesia, surgery, and life-threatening allergic reactions: epidemiology and clinical features of perioperative anaphylaxis in the 6th National Audit Project (NAP6). *Br J Anaesth*, **121(1):** 159–71.

30. Robinson, M. and Davidson, A. (2014) Aspiration under anaesthesia: risk assessment and decision-making. *Contin Educ Anaesth Crit Care Pain*, **14(4):** 17–5.

31. Ray, K., Bodenham, A. and Paramasivam, E. (2014) Pulmonary atelectasis in anaesthesia and critical care. *Contin Educ Anaesth Crit Care Pain*, **14(5):** 236–45.

32. Lee, J.I. and Ahn, H.J. (2010) General anesthesia in a patient with known bronchial anthracofibrosis – a case report. *Korean J Anesthesiol*, **58(3):** 307–10.

33. Hardman, J.G. and Aitkenhead, A.R. (2005) Awareness during anaesthesia. *Contin Educ Anaesth Crit Care Pain*, **5(6):** 183–6.

34. Pandit, J.J., Andrade, J., Bogod, D.G. *et al.* (2014) 5th National Audit Project (NAP5) on accidental awareness during general anaesthesia: summary of main findings and risk factors. *Br J Anaesth*, **113(4):** 549–59.

35. Looseley, A. (2011) Management of bronchospasm during general anaesthesia. *Update in Anaesthesia*, **27(1):** 17–21.

36. Gavel, G. and Walker, R.W. (2013) Laryngospasm in anaesthesia. *Contin Educ Anaesth Crit Care Pain*, **14(2):** 47–51.

37. Schneiderbanger, D., Johannsen, S., Roewer, N. and Schuster, F. (2014) Management of malignant hyperthermia: diagnosis and treatment. *Ther Clin Risk Manag*, **10:** 355–62.

38. Rees, J. (2003) Suxamethonium apnoea. *Update in Anaesthesia*.

39. Lopez, M.B. (2018) Postanaesthetic shivering – from pathophysiology to prevention. *Rom J Anaesth Intensive Care*, **25(1):** 73–81.

40. Chang, A. and White, B.A. (2020) *Peripheral Nerve Blocks*. StatPearls.

41. Dangle, J., Kukreja, P. and Kalagara, H. (2020) Review of current practices of peripheral nerve blocks for hip fracture and surgery. *Current Anesthesiology Reports*, **10(3):** 259–66.

42. Newman, B. (2010) *Complete Spinal Block Following Spinal Anaesthesia*. Anaesthesia tutorial of week 180. World Federation of Societies of Anaesthesiologists.

43. Kwak, K.H. (2017) Postdural puncture headache. *Korean J Anesthesiol*, **70(2):** 136–4.

44. Ankcorn, C. (2000) Spinal anaesthesia – a practical guide. *Update in Anaesthesia*.

45. Cook, T.M., Counsell, D., Wildsmith, J.A. and Royal College of Anaesthetists Third National Audit Project (2009) Major complications of central neuraxial block: report on the Third National Audit Project of the Royal College of Anaesthetists. *Br J Anaesth*, **102(2):** 179–90.

46. Pierre, S. and Whelan, R. (2012) Nausea and vomiting after surgery. *Contin Educ Anaesth Crit Care Pain*, **13(1)**: 28–32.

47. Apfel, C.C., Heidrich, F.M., Jukar-Rao, S. *et al.* (2012) Evidence-based analysis of risk factors for postoperative nausea and vomiting. *Br J Anaesth*, **109(5):** 742–53.

48. Dewinter, G., Staelens, W., Veef, E. *et al.* (2018) Simplified algorithm for the prevention of postoperative nausea and vomiting: a before-and-after study. *Br J Anaesth*, **120(1):** 156–63.

49. Shaikh, S.I, Nagarekha, D., Hegade, G. and Marutheesh, M. (2016) Postoperative nausea and vomiting: a simple yet complex problem. *Anesth Essays Res*, **10(3):** 388–396.

50. Dagi, T.F. (2005) The management of postoperative bleeding. *Surg Clin North Am*, **85(6):** 1191–213.

51. Pomajzl, A.J. and Siref, L.E. (2020) *Post-op Urinary Retention*. StatPearls.

52. NICE (2019, updated 2020) *Surgical site infections: prevention and treatment* [NG125]. Available from: www.nice.org.uk/guidance/NG125.

53. Hasselmann, J. (2019) Prevention of surgical wound complications after peripheral vascular surgery. PhD Thesis.

54. Murrell, Z.A. and Stamos, M.J. (2006) Reoperation for anastomotic failure. *Clin Colon Rectal Surg*, **19(4):** 213–6.

55. NICE (2020) *Venous thromboembolic diseases: diagnosis, management and thrombophilia testing* [NG158]. Available from: www.nice.org.uk/guidance/NG158.

56. Wells, P.S., Anderson, D.R., Rodger, M. *et al.* (2003) Evaluation of D-dimer in the diagnosis of suspected deep-vein thrombosis. *N Engl J Med*, **349(13):** 1227–35.

57. Kasturi, S. (2021) Current concepts in the diagnosis and management of pulmonary embolism. *International Journal of Clinical Medicine*, **12:** 115–29.

58. NICE (2019, updated 2022) *Scenario: Suspected pulmonary embolism*. Available from: https://cks.nice.org.uk/topics/pulmonary-embolism/management/suspected-pulmonary-embolism.

Figure acknowledgements

Figure 1.1 Supplied by the authors.

Figure 1.2 Reproduced from Richardson, R. and Ellis, R. (2022) *Clinical Specialties: medical student revision guide*. Scion Publishing Ltd.

Figure 1.3 Adapted from Marshall, P., Gallacher, B., Jolly, J. and Rinomhota, S. (2017) *Anatomy and Physiology in Healthcare*. Scion Publishing Ltd.

Figure 2.2 Reproduced from https://commons.wikimedia.org/w/index.php?curid=12842847 under a CC BY-SA 3.0 licence. Author: Jmarchn.

Figure 2.4 Reproduced from https://commons.wikimedia.org/wiki/File:Knee-high_and_thigh-high_anti-embolism_compression_stockings.jpg under a Creative Commons Attribution-Share Alike 4.0 International licence. Author: Lentpjuve.

Figure 2.5 Reproduced from Dennis, M., Sandercock, P., Reid, J. *et al.* (2013) Effectiveness of intermittent pneumatic compression in reduction of risk of deep vein thrombosis in patients who have had a stroke (CLOTS 3): a multicentre randomised controlled trial. *The Lancet*, **382(9891)**, with permission from Elsevier.

Figure 3.1 Reproduced from Sellers, C. and Woodman, N. (2023) Inhalational induction in paediatric anaesthesia. *BJA Education*, **23(1):** 32-8, with permission from Elsevier.

Figure 3.2 Reproduced from Tsukamoto, M., Taura, S., Yamanaka, H. *et al.* (2020) Age-related effects of three inhalational anesthetics at one minimum alveolar concentration on electroencephalogram waveform. *Aging Clin Exp Res*, **32(9):** 1857–64, Springer Nature.

Figure 4.2 Reproduced under a Creative Commons Licence (with adaptation) from Elbaih, A.H. B.F. (2020) Teaching approach of primary survey in trauma patients. *International Journal of Internal and Emergency Medicine*, **3(3):** 1035.

Figure 4.3 Used with permission of MA Healthcare Ltd, from Sampson, M. (2021) A guide to airway management. *British Journal of Cardiac Nursing*, **16(3):** 1–13; permission conveyed through Copyright Clearance Center, Inc.

Figure 4.4 Reproduced from Richardson, R. and Keeling, J. (2021) *Clinical Skills: an introduction for nursing and healthcare*, with permission from Lantern Publishing Ltd.

Figure 4.5 Reproduced from Goudra, B. and Singh, P.M. (2017) Airway management during upper GI endoscopic procedures: state of the art review. *Dig Dis Sci*, **62(1):** 45–53, with permission from Springer Nature.

Figure 4.6 Reproduced from Santillanes, G. and Gausche-Hill, M. (2008) Pediatric airway management. *Emerg Med Clin N Am*, **26(4):** 961–975, with permission from Elsevier.

Figure 4.7 Reproduced from Smith, S.L. and Thomson, S.L. (2013) Influence of subglottic stenosis on the flow-induced vibration of a computational vocal fold model. *J Fluids Struct*, **38:** 77–91.

Figure 4.8 Reproduced from https://commons.wikimedia.org/wiki/File:Laryngeal_mask_airway.jpg under a Creative Commons Attribution-Share Alike 4.0 International licence. Author: ICUnurses.

Figure 4.10 Reproduced with permission from Intersurgical Ltd.

Figure 4.11 Reproduced from *Equipment in Anaesthesia and Critical Care*. Scion Publishing Ltd.

Figure 4.12 Reproduced from Ruetzler, K., Smereka, J., Abelairas-Gomez, C. *et al.* (2020) Comparison of the new flexible tip bougie catheter and standard bougie stylet for tracheal intubation by anesthesiologists in different difficult airway scenarios: a randomized crossover trial. *BMC Anesthesiology*, **20(1):** 90 under a CC Attribution 4.0 International Licence.

Figure 4.13 Reproduced from Ruetzler, K., Szarpak, L., Smereka, J. *et al.* (2020) Comparison of direct and video laryngoscopes during different airway scenarios performed by experienced paramedics: a randomized cross-over manikin study. *BioMed Research International*, 5382739 under the CC Attribution Licence.

Figure 4.14 Reproduced under a CC BY-SA 3.0 licence from https://commons.wikimedia.org/wiki/File:Larynx_endo_2.jpg#/media/File:Larynx_endo_2.jpg. Author: Samir.

Figure 4.15 Reproduced from Ansari, L., Bohluli, B., Mahaseni, H. *et al.* (2014) The effect of endotracheal tube cuff pressure control on postextubation throat pain in orthognathic surgeries: a randomized double-blind controlled clinical trial. *British Journal of Oral and Maxillofacial Surgery*, **52(2):** 140–143, with permission from Elsevier.

Figure 4.16 Reproduced with permission from the Difficult Airway Society.

Figure 5.1 Reproduced from Lee, J.I. and Ahn, H.J. (2010) General anesthesia in a patient with known bronchial anthracofibrosis – a case report. *Korean J Anesthesiol*, **58(3):** 307–10.

Figure 7.1 Reproduced from Dangle, J., Kukreja, P. and Kalagara, H. (2020) Review of current practices of peripheral nerve blocks for hip fracture and surgery. *Curr Anesthesiol Rep*, **10:** 259–266.

Figure 7.3 Reproduced under a Creative Commons Attribution 4.0 International License from https://commons.wikimedia.org/wiki/File:Epidural-anesthesia.png. Authors: Leila Kafshdooz, Houman Kahroba, Tayebeh Kafshdooz, Roghayeh Sheervalilou & Hojjat Pourfathi.

Figure 7.4 Reproduced under a Creative Commons Attribution-Share Alike 3.0 Unported licence from https://commons.wikimedia.org/wiki/File:Prinzip_der_Spinalanaesthesie.en.svg

Figure 8.1 Reproduced from Hasselmann, J. (2019) Prevention of surgical wound complications after peripheral vascular surgery. PhD Thesis, with permission.

Figure 8.2 Reproduced under a Creative Commons Attribution-Share Alike 3.0 Unported licence from https://commons.wikimedia.org/wiki/File:Deep_vein_thrombosis_of_the_right_leg.jpg. Author: James Heilman, MD.

Figure 8.3 Reproduced from Kasturi, S. (2021) Current concepts in the diagnosis and management of pulmonary embolism. *International Journal of Clinical Medicine*, **12:** 115–129, under a Creative Commons Attribution 4.0 International licence.

Index

Bold indicates main entry

Acetylcholinesterase, 14, **85**
Addison's disease, 33–4
Adrenaline, 2, 74, 80, 89–90
Airway adjuncts, 59–61
   head tilt–chin lift, 57, 59
   jaw thrust, 57–9, 62
   nasopharyngeal airways, 59, 60, 63
   oropharyngeal airways, 58, 59
Allergy, 45, 74, 96, 98
American Society of Anesthesiologists' (ASA)
   classification, 25–8
Amino-steroid drug, 16
Anaesthetic history, 21
Analgesia
   aspirin, 35, 42
   codeine, 11, 102
   dihydrocodeine, 11
   fentanyl, 99
   gabapentin, 11
   ibuprofen, 11
   magnesium sulphate, 61
   Oramorph, 12
   paracetamol, 11, 102
   pregabalin, 11
   tramadol, 12
Anaphylaxis, 16, 74, 80
Anastomotic leak, 116–17
Angioedema, 74
Antacids, 37
Antibiotics, 45, 74, 113–17
Anticoagulant, 35, 42, 103, 120
Antiembolism stockings, 40–2
Anti-emetic, 108–9
Anxiolytics, 37
Apfel score, 108–9
Apixaban, 42, 120
Aspiration pneumonia, 76, 113–15
Atelectasis, **77–8**, 113, 115
   absorption, 77
   compression, 77
Atlanto-axial subluxation, 30
Atrial fibrillation, 121
Autonomic gastroparesis, 50
Awareness during general anaesthesia, 79
   explicit, 79
   implicit, 79
Axillary approach to the brachial
   plexus, 97

Battle's sign, 61
Benzodiazepines, 7, 37
Benzylisoquinolinium, 16–17
Bladder scan, 112
Blood
   cultures, 102, 113–14
   products, 29–31, 110–11
Brachial plexus, 97
Bronchoscopy, 76
Bronchospasm, 17, 74, **80–1**
Bupivacaine, 88, **90**, 98, 104

Calcium, 84, 120
Cancer, 42, 119–20, 121–2
Capnography, 52, 63, 68, 80, 84
Cardiac steal syndrome, 9
Cardiac ventricles, 121
Carotid endarterectomy, 97
Cerebrospinal fluid (CSF), 61
Cervical plexus block, 97
Chlorhexidine, 115
Chlorphenamine, 74
Clotting profile, 26–9, 35, 41
Co-amoxiclav, 115
Collection, 113, 117
Compound A, 9
C-reactive protein (CRP), 102, 114, 117
Cricoid cartilage, 50, 65
Cricoid pressure, 50
Cross-match, 29, 30
Crystalloid, 111
CSF rhinorrhoea, 61
CT pulmonary angiogram, 123
Cyclizine, 109

Dantrolene, 84
D-dimer test, 119–20, 123
Deep vein thrombosis (DVT), **38–41**, 117–23
Dentition, 24
Dexamethasone, 109
Diabetes, 26–9, 32–3
Doppler USS, 119
Dural puncture, 101–3

Emergency front of neck access (FONA), 71
End of anaesthesia, 53
   enhanced recovery after surgery
     (ERAS), 53

Enoxaprin, 35, 42, 119, 123
Epidural anaesthesia, 98–103
Epidural haematoma, 103
Epidural space, 88, **99–101**, 103
Epigastric, 68
Epiglottis, 67, 70
Epilepsy, 5–6, 36
Epistaxis, 60
Ester hydrolysis, 17
Expiratory wheeze, 80
Exploratory laparotomy, 117

Fascial planes, 88, 95
Fasciculations, 13, **15–16**
Fasting, 44, 50, 75
Fat embolism, 121
Femoral nerve, 97
Fleischner sign, 122
Foramen magnum, 100
Full blood count (FBC), 26–8, 102, 114

Group and save, 29, 30
Guedel airway, 58

Haemoptysis, 122
Haemorrhage
   primary, 110–11
   secondary, 110–11
Haemotympanum, 61
Halothane, 10
Hampton hump, 122
HbA1c, 29
Hepatitis, 10
High dependency unit (HDU), 43
Hoarseness, 69
Hofmann elimination, 17
Homans sign, 118
Hospital-acquired pneumonia, 113–14
Hydrocortisone, 33, 74
Hyperthermia, malignant, 15, 22, 54, **84**
Hypnosis, 2–3, 6
Hypnotic agents, 4, 7, 52
Hypothermia, 8, **86**

Iliac crest, 104
Iliohypogastric nerve, 97
Ilioinguinal nerve, 97
Ilioinguinal/iliohypogastric nerve block, 97
Immobilisation, 36, 118–19, 122
Induction anaesthesia, 49
   gaseous induction, 49, 51–2
   rapid sequence induction, 15, **50**
Inspiratory stridor, 82
Insulin, 2, 32–3
Intensive care unit (ICU), 43

Intermittent pneumatic compression
      devices, 41
International normalised ratio (INR), 35,
      42, 120
Interscalene block, 97
Intervertebral space, 103
Intralipid, 92
Ischaemic bowel, 117
Isoflurane, 8–9

Ketamine, 7

Lactate, 117
Laparotomy, exploratory, 117
Laryngospasm, 82–3
Lateral femoral cutaneous nerve, 97
Levofloxacin, 115
Lidocaine, 5, 88, **89**
Ligamentum flavum, 99
Local anaesthesia, 88–92
Low molecular weight heparin (LMWH), 35, 42
Lumbar plexus, 97
Lumbosacral plexus block, 97

Macintosh laryngoscope, 67
Magnesium sulphate, 81
Maintenance anaesthesia, 51–2
   bispectral EEG, 51
   total intravenous anaesthesia (TIVA), **51–2**,
      109
Malignant hyperthermia, 15, 22, 54, **84**
Mallampati score, 23
Mammogram, 120
Masseter spasm, 84
Mast cell tryptase, 74
Median nerve, 97
Metformin, 32
Metronidazole, 115
Minimum alveolar concentration, 8
Musculocutaneous nerve, 97
Myasthenia gravis, 17, 18

Nausea, see Postoperative nausea and
      vomiting (PONV)
Neuraxial techniques, 94, **98**, 104
Neuromuscular blockers, **13–14**, 17
   atracurium, 17
   rocuronium, 16–18
   suxamethonium, 15, 85
Neuromuscular junction, **13–14**, 17
Nicotinic receptors, **13–14**
Nil by mouth, 117; see also Fasting

Obturator nerve, 97
Oesophageal intubation, 68–9

Ondansetron, 109
Opiate, 11, 99, 131, 133
Oral contraceptive pill, 36, 39

Pain ladder, 11–12
Parkinson's disease, 36, 50
Patient-controlled epidural analgesia, 100
Percutaneous drainage, 117
Peripheral nerve block, 88, 94, **95–6**
Plasma cholinesterases, 15
Pneumonia, 76, **113–15**
Pneumothorax, 70
Popliteal nerve block, 97
Positive pressure ventilation, 77
Post-dural puncture headache (PDPH), 102
Postoperative nausea and vomiting (PONV),
52, 94, **108–9**
Postoperative urinary retention (POUR),
111–12
Prednisolone, 33
Preoperative assessment clinic (POAC), 20
Propofol, **5**, 49, 51
infusion syndrome, 5
Pulmonary embolism, 121–3
Pyrexia, **113–15**, 121

QT interval, 52

Raccoon eyes, 61
Radial nerve, 97

Sciatic nerve block, 97
Sepsis, **113**, 114, 117
Sevoflurane, 9
SGLT-2 inhibitors, 32
Shower, 115
Sign-in, 45
Sign-out, 46
Spinal anaesthesia, 98–9, **104–5**
Sputum, 114
Staphylococcus aureus, 115
Sternomental distance, 24
Stridor, 65, 82
inspiratory, 82
Stroke, 123
Subglottic airway devices/procedures, 65–72
bougie, 66, 68, 70
cricothyroidotomy, 69–71
endotracheal tube, 50, **65–9**, 70, 81
intubation, 50, **65–71**

laryngoscope, 66–9
tracheostomy, 69–71
video-assisted laryngoscope, 68
Subglottic stenosis, 65, 70
Suggamadex, 16
Sulphonylurea, 32
Supraglottic airway devices, **62–4**, 71
i-gel airway, 64
laryngeal mask airway, **62–3**, 71, 76
Surgical grade, 25–6, 29
Surgical site infection, 113, **115–16**
Surgical stress response, 2, 4, 11, 32–3
Suxamethonium apnoea
(pseudocholinesterase deficiency), 15,
22, **85**
Swabs, 29, 46, 116
Systematic vascular resistance, 5–6, 9, 105

Temporomandibular joint, 24
Theophylline, 81
Thiopental sodium (aka thiopentone), 6
Thrombectomy, 123
Thrombolysis, 123
Thyromental distance, 24
Time out, 45
Tonsillectomy, 25, 82
Total spinal anaesthesia, 101, 105
Transversus abdominus plane block, 97
Triad of anaesthesia, **3–4**

Ulnar nerve, 97
Unanticipated difficult airway, 68, 70, 72
Urinary retention, 105, 111–12
Urine output, 110, 113, 117

Vallecula, 67–8
Venous thromboembolism (VTE), **38–42**, 117,
123
Ventilation/perfusion scan (V/Q scan), 123
Vertebrae, 30, 50, 100, 104
Video laryngoscopy, 30, 68, 70
Virchow's triad, 38, 40
Volatile agents, 8
Vomiting, *see* Postoperative nausea and
vomiting (PONV)

Warfarin, 35, 42, 120
Wells score, 119, 122–3
Westermark sign, 122
World Health Organization, 11, 45, 46